Inside Youth Sports

Inside Youth Sports

An Expert's and Athlete's Guide to Health, Fitness, Competition and Better Play

Buel D. Rodgers, PhD, and Meilani Y. Rodgers

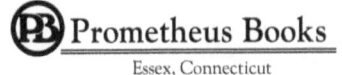
Prometheus Books
Essex, Connecticut

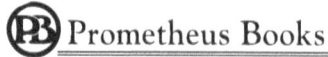 Prometheus Books

An imprint of The Globe Pequot Publishing Group, Inc.
64 South Main St.
Essex, CT 06426
www.GlobePequot.com

Copyright © 2026 by Buel D. Rodgers, Ph.D. and Meilani Y. Rodgers

All rights reserved. No part of this book may be reproduced in any form or by any electronic or mechanical means, including information storage and retrieval systems, without written permission from the publisher, except by a reviewer who may quote passages in a review.

British Library Cataloguing in Publication Information available

Library of Congress Cataloging-in-Publication Data available

ISBN 978-1-4930-9836-1 (cloth)
ISBN 978-1-4930-9122-5 (paperback)
ISBN 978-1-4930-9224-6 (ebook)

Contents

Chapter 1: Pregame 1

Chapter 2: The Gift 7

Chapter 3: Body and Mind 21

Chapter 4: The Metamorphosis 45

Chapter 5: Pink or Blue? 73

Chapter 6: Bowling Balls, Meat Cleavers and Chainsaws 91

Chapter 7: Toto, I've a Feeling We're Not in Idaho Anymore 119

Chapter 8: Killing Coyotes 137

Chapter 9: Mount Rushmore 159

Chapter 10: Plot Twists 189

Chapter 11: The ACL Problem 213

Chapter 12: Postgame 223

Notes 233

Index 237

Chapter 1

Pregame

I'm a dad. I'm a dad who loves to play. I'm a dad who loves sports and, most of all, loves playing sports with his kids. I'm also a dad who lives vicariously through their lives, possibly too much and too often, although I try my best to respect their boundaries and admit feeling insecure in this role. Children are born into boundaries, physical boundaries at first, taking the form of receiving blankets, bassinets, carriers, bouncers and cribs, all of which are replaced by more ephemeral boundaries as they age, like rules and regulations or societal norms for play and expression. They even begin creating their own boundaries especially as adolescents, exploring their self-proclaimed freedoms and testing those assigned by parents and other authorities. Child athletes are particularly immersed in boundaries. Who, what, when, where, why and how they play are all controlled by parents, coaches and league or school regulations, not the athlete who ironically is the most susceptible to the system's flaws or authority figures' sins.

Should child athletes control their fate? Should they possess veto power over what sport they play, what team they join, when they practice or compete, how often and how aggressive or seriously they play? Quite frankly, no, at least not entirely. A child's health and wellbeing are hardly their responsibility because children are hardly capable of being responsible. We as parents aren't willing to abdicate control of our children's intellectual development so doing so with their physical development

Chapter 1

is hypocritical if not nonsensical. Should child athletes have a voice in making important decisions, should their opinions always be considered? Yes, emphatically! "Considered," however, is not unambiguous and all too often patronizing, at least when parents or coaches feign to empower their children and athletes with lip service.

Consider the analogy of clinical drug trials for rare terminal diseases as, for example, with Duchenne muscular dystrophy or "DMD." This crippling muscle wasting disease has no cure and a median life expectancy of only 22 years, although subjects with more severe forms die as adolescents. Parents desperate to help their children compete for clinical trial slots yet their fate is not determined at random, by themselves or even by their child. It's determined by strict inclusion criteria previously developed by medical and scientific experts, reviewed by two or even three institutional review boards or "IRBs" and approved by the Food and Drug Administration. The decision of inclusion is *made in the best interest of the patient* and is completely insensitive to the patient's or parents' desires. Likewise, a child athlete's voice should be respected, although ultimately parents make the decision and this must absolutely be based on the child athlete's *needs* rather than *wants*.

My daughter and I wrote this book because we both struggled in distinguishing our *needs* from *wants*. In fact, both changed as she matriculated through the competitive youth sports arena, further obscuring the line of distinction. We presumed others might be interested in our perspectives that are in some ways very typical and in others very unique. I myself am an athlete. I'm also a scientist, inventor, coach, mentor and teacher. Like most people, I wear many hats and like most hats, some fit better than others. My childhood dream was to play in the "majors," third base for the Cincinnati Reds who as it turns out weren't that interested in a 140-pound infielder with average arm strength, an uncanny skill for bunting but an inability to hit the curve. The truth is that I was never a particularly good athlete, average at best you might say, yet my greatest "what if" in life is never seriously pursuing my true athletic talent until I was too busy to devote, too committed to dedicate and, let's face it, too old to accomplish. I nevertheless milked the most from the fields, tracks and roads where I played and as a result, grew as a person and even as a scientist.

Pregame

For 30 years and counting I've been conducting research in the field of muscle development, earning a PhD from the University of California, Berkeley, and working at the National Institute on Aging, the Johns Hopkins University School of Medicine and Washington State University. My understanding of muscle biology and exercise science is reflected in the scientific literature, in several patents and in textbook chapters. I've shared this knowledge in lectures to fellow scientists at various stages of career development and in my training of postdoctoral and medical fellows, graduate and undergraduate students and technicians. I've also won multiple awards for research, teaching and mentoring and was appointed to prestigious committees and leadership positions in what would have been an illustrious career in academia, that is until my parents, a niece and nephew were diagnosed with terminal muscle wasting diseases. Both parents died shortly after being diagnosed while the others, as of this writing, survive in disability to their condition.

The irony of my family's fate and my chosen profession is inescapable. It is also motivational. Rather than continue in a field dominated by the esoteric, with few rewards outside an occasional ego stroking, I left academia to start a biotech company that develops gene therapeutics for muscle wasting disorders. The decision came as an epiphany, while angrily composing a response to an imbecile reviewer lording control over my manuscript's fate, feigning competence and unknowingly compelling me into an alternative career path. Yes, I recognize I have an ego and no, I don't truly believe this person was an imbecile, but the experience reminded me of Sayre's law, albeit slightly revised: "Academic egos are so large because the stakes are so low." The "stakes" are indeed high in my family and the banality of arguing with an anonymous academic, with academia in general, no longer held any appeal so I held my breath and jumped.

My belabored point is that I understand the science of exercise better than every coach I've ever met and with all humility, better than most professional coaches. In fact, professional teams hire specialized strength and conditioning coaches and physical therapists precisely because most coaches lack this knowledge. Such specialists possess a practical understanding of exercise science that is far superior to my own and when combined with motivational and sport-science expertise creates a mentoring environment optimized for the professional athlete. My understanding of muscle physiology and exercise science is more academic yet deep and intimate. It is derived from laboratory experiments with muscle stem cells, with animal models of different muscle diseases like DMD or cancer cachexia and from using exercise routines or "VO_2 max tests" to measure oxygen consumption during high-intensity exercise, all to better understand muscle disease and to develop novel drugs. It stems from studying the biomechanics of running, the excitation-contraction coupling of individual cardiac muscle cells and the biological generation of *power* or *work*, specific terms of my trade, when isolated muscles are connected to a force transducer. My research sought to define the fundamentals, how muscle grows and how it evolved, as well as the applied, how it can be repaired.

An understanding of exercise science is of course only a single arrow in the coaching quiver. Coaches are teachers and mentors, managers of expertise and experiences. Their goals and responsibilities change with the age and accomplishment of their athletes, or at least they should. I would argue that many of our concerns over coaching and youth sports are rooted not in poor or overzealous coaching but in the mismatch of coaching priorities and style of play with those of their athletes. I too have coached, quite a bit actually. Starting with my son's youth baseball teams and later as my daughter's running coach and a high school track coach, although like a surgeon who can't or shouldn't operate on loved ones, I recognized the importance of deferring my authority to other coaches whose talents were sometimes superior and sometimes inferior to my own, at least in the traditional coaching role.

I made mistakes as a coach, not so much with other kids but with my own. One of my former baseball players might object to getting beaned four times in just one batting session (sorry Hayden), but I assure you and him that the 12 year old learned to turn away from the assault precisely because I hit him, not intentionally of course. Mistakes are natural to any learning process and with every beaned child or accidental outburst or overlooked injury, I adapted, changed and improved. I also learned just how difficult coaching can be even for someone with an understanding of exercise science, who has won multiple teaching and mentoring awards and who himself loves to play. This is because coaching requires patience as much as knowledge, empathy as much as desire and sacrifice as much as skill. It is also especially difficult to do when children and their families are involved.

As a coach and as a parent, I lived for and through my children's experiences. I suspect we all do. We want what's best for them and by proxy for ourselves. It's not selfish, it's Darwinian. It's also incredibly important to recognize the vicariousness of our relationships and its potential risk to our children's emotional, intellectual and physical development as well as to their safe journey to independence.

Many of the chapters ahead are co-written by my daughter and me, starting with my contribution and concluding with "Meilani's Take," an adolescent's first-person perspectives written at different ages. They record both good and bad experiences, among which are objective assessments of the youth sports juggernaut, the community of coaches, athletes and families as well as an occasional humorous anecdote and overly detailed dive into the minutia. They also provide professional guidance and how-tos, proactive advice for navigating the youth sporting experience that's backed by informed science and healthcare knowledge and validated by quite possibly the two most successful college coaches in history, "GOATs" for their respective sports. We discuss real people and real events, from our own biased perspective of course, and use fictitious names from literature to protect identities, begrudgingly in some cases and with a little tongue-in-cheek jocularity. The identities of paid coaches, however, are either preserved in positive review as a reward for embodying authoritative coaching or are protected. Our goal is to educate and reform, not to requite, yet I suspect few of the derelict are capable of self-reflection.

Most importantly, we readily admit our own subjectivities, defend our objectivities and advocate critical thinking when discussing both personal experiences and established dogma. The latter include science, which features prominently in many chapters and especially when discussing exercise physiology, the physical and mental benefits of exercise, the assessment of coaching trends and approaches, sports' impact on

Chapter 1

puberty and vice versa as well as possibly the most controversial contemporary topic of youth sports: transgender athletes.

Who is our audience? Well, for one it's parents of athletic children. It's also former youth athletes, amateur and professional youth coaches, school athletic coordinators and league organizers. Most importantly, it's the families of adolescent athletes, some of whom might consider playing at "the next level" or who have "D1 aspirations." These clichés are repeated incessantly, often with sincerity by recruiters, coaches and parents with discerning standards yet just as often by recruiters, coaches and parents who lack either sincerity or standards. Some may even be malicious in their praise, narcissistically manipulating athletes and their families for financial or emotional gain. It's genuinely difficult to tell and to be honest, I'm not convinced it matters, as long as parents and athletes alike focus on the most laudable goal of competitive play and organized sports: personal growth. The rest will follow, honestly, it really will.

Chapter 2

The Gift

She's gifted. She really is. That amorphic thing separating her from her peers, at least in athletics. She has "*IT*."

I remember holding my breath the first time I saw her really run, as hard and as fast as she could, tempted and challenged by boys and girls her age, some even a couple years older. Yes, I know what you're thinking, "How cliché," but I really did hold my breath. I had seen her run many times before, but not among a crowd and only with her brother or a few friends. I knew she was fast and I knew my love of running had influenced her. I even suspected she ran to please "Dada," but this was different. She was running among her peers, in a competitive environment and all around her were sloths.

I remember a feeling of awe, staring at something both foreign and familiar. Was this really my little girl? Gliding effortlessly, gracefully, powerfully across the field and with perfect form nonetheless, overtaking kids twice her size, boys and girls alike.

I remember being surprised by my admiration. Not by a feeling of joy, but of both pride and jealousy. My 7-year-old daughter ran better than I did. Despite several decades of running experience and a professional understanding of running biomechanics and muscle dynamics, my daughter, in all her frailty and silliness, ran with less effort and more refined strength than I ever had. Her form was absolutely perfect. No jerky motions. Arms quickly pumping, hands moving from hips to shoulders, straight and without any lateral movements. She ran on the "front" of her stride, stepping as soon as her knee passed her hip, propelling her forward with absolutely no vertical movement, shin parallel to the ground, heals tracking straight to her butt and never touching the ground.

Parents commented, "Wow, look at her! How long has she been playing? Who's been coaching her?"

I was an avid runner and well recognized in the community, not only from university outreach events and coaching youth baseball but from running the small town streets and backcountry roads. Most parents probably assumed that I had coached her, but I hadn't, not yet. In fact, her closest coaching experience with anyone probably came from watching baseball, which she did solely to get Dada's attention and that hasn't changed. Her running form was innate, genetic, natural. It was also on full display.

It was an incredibly beautiful morning, as it usually is on clear days in the Pacific Northwest. The air was cool and crisp and everything seemed to reflect the sun's morning yellow. Mountainview Park was at the edge of Moscow, surrounded by wheat fields with Moscow Mountain overlooking from the north and set against a stunning sapphire blue sky. Young children filled the field wearing brightly colored sweatpants, tights or baggy shorts with sweatshirts or black-and-gold rec jerseys, scurrying across a green canvas of grass.

Mei was at first a little nervous, reticent to join the few scattered groups lazily kicking the ball around. She hadn't yet recognized any of the other kids and stood quietly by my side. I encouraged her to join the fun, but she preferred to wait until the coach arrived. Such nervousness is natural and as I looked around, I discovered it was also the norm. More kids arrived and more stood quietly next to their parents.

"Microsoccer" was more about socializing than learning the game. Learning occurs through a progression, one that is built upon a foundation of rules, not in the classic definition, but guiding principles of thought and in this case play. Kids needed to first learn that the coach was now in charge, not them nor their parents. They needed to learn to feel safe and protected and that their trust would be reciprocated. They needed to learn that trying alone would be awarded and failure would be encouraged. They needed to learn that criticism would not be tolerated unless of course they broke the rules. The goal was to build appreciation for play, for the team, for the experience and for oneself, which in my mind is the true beauty of sports.

Once all this is established, then the rules of the game could be taught before moving on to the more complicated task of learning skills. In its most elementary form, soccer may be a simple game of kick and run, yet even this can be difficult to teach when the learning environment is compromised by a misbehaving child or corrupted by an interrupting yet well-meaning parent. In fact, dealing with misbehaving child athletes or even worse, their misbehaving parents is by far the most frustrating and anxiety-inducing aspect of coaching youth sports, and although children can be easily controlled or redirected, their parents cannot.

My most challenging coaching experiences were always a result of parental interference. The worst situations occurred during practice or involved coaches who were also the parent of a player. Practice environments usually occur in the absence of a discerning audience, for example, other parents or league staff that would normally condemn poor behavior. This forces coaches to either confront the abuser in "mano-a-mano" fashion or to report the abuse. For several reasons, good coaches recognize the need to do both. Parents are susceptible to pressure from below, meaning from their own kids, and players are less likely to act out when they witness a superior (i.e., an adult) be disciplined. Most importantly, league managers have the ability to ban parents from official league events including practices and games. I suspect some leagues are reluctant to invoke such "nuclear options" out of fear that it indirectly punishes the child. Hogwash! Removing the abuser protects *all* the children and sends a very clear message to other wannabe abusers: cross the line and you're gone.

I once had a parent who constantly denigrated his son. He attended every practice and game and shouted insults at every opportunity, which of course only made his son play even worse. When tactfully asked to stop, the father responded with, "Yeah that's not gonna happen." The other coach and I tried in vain over several practices and games, probably too many, to get him to behave. We finally contacted league authorities and the problem was solved with a single phone call.

Without his father's incessant berating, the boy's confidence immediately improved as did his performance. We eventually invited his father back to practice and then to help as a volunteer, a "distract and empower" approach that works equally well with players who lack developed attention spans. You can't imagine how many times I feigned accidents, spilling whole buckets of baseballs only to solicit my favorite players' help in picking them up. Most kids thought I was clumsy and funny, some understood and said nothing while the attention seekers just thought I needed help. They were also elated to provide it.

My point is to emphasize the importance of establishing and maintaining a proper learning environment. After all, nobody would accept a child or adult screaming in the middle of math class, but for some reason we tolerate it at youth sporting events. Quickly establishing the rules of learning as well as the consequences for violating these rules is paramount to coaching. It applies to every sport, to every age and to every person involved including fellow coaches, players, parents and spectators.

Mei's first soccer coach understood this lesson well. She, the coach, played soccer in college and had coached for only a few years but applied a commonsense motherly approach that quickly established a foundation for learning. She held the first practice just before the first game, which at this age was more of an abstract concept than an organized event. Goals weren't counted, outcomes weren't recorded and for the most part, everyone was well behaved outside of an occasional stop to pick up dandelions or to turn a cartwheel. Such cavalier play is blasphemous in some parts of the country, but in a Northern Idaho college town, it was welcomed by parents more interested in their barista's gossip than in the sanctity of sport.

Each team had eight players, four on the field and four neatly sitting along the sideline, their butts absorbing the morning dew. The "starters" were randomly picked and placed by their respective coaches in 1-2-1 diamond formations, a single "forward" in the front followed by two "mids" hugging the outside lines and a "defender" in the back. The referee called the two forwards to the ball, explained how the game began and then blew the whistle.

Mei exploded down the line, flew past the other team and stopped in front of the goal. She was already hopping up and down yelling for the ball before the referee could restart the game. Her teammate, lost in the moment, had forgotten the instructions and kicked the ball forward against the rules. Parents laughed, the players returned to their positions, the referee once again blew the whistle . . . and history repeated itself two more times.

The kids eventually figured it out and by the season's end had transitioned from an unbridled peloton of legs flinging the ball in random directions to somewhat organized play, spread out with passing, dribbling and marginally accurate shooting. Mei would score 10 or 12 goals playing just half of a 20-minute game. She was faster and more aggressive than anyone she played with or against and it was clear, even from such an early age, that recreational soccer wouldn't satisfy her competitive hunger.

Travel soccer was a much better fit for her appetite and she relished playing among the structure and commitment of the Moscow United Soccer Club. She also continued to thrive as the team's scoring champion; multi-goal games were the norm and "hat tricks" were a regularity. She devoured anything soccer, participating in every soccer and futsal camp available and almost always winning a camp award, although ironically soccer wasn't her best sport.

Mei was destined to run track. Her stride had always been more art than mechanics and although we wanted to avoid the well-documented risks of early sports specialization, we questioned whether she'd rejoice or recoil with the change. The sport lacks appeal to many young athletes and this is especially true for distance events. It's also true for children who prefer, desire or require strong social interactions to thrive, which soccer handsomely provided, or even to enjoy an experience. Mei has always been a social beast, blind to age, sex or any other demographic and she considered group interactions as opportunities to make friends. For this reason we were reluctant to introduce a sport that demanded so much personal commitment and individual effort. Then we met Coach Mike.

Chapter 2

Mike Hinz coached the Comets Track Club in Pullman, Washington, for over 30 years. He was also the head coach for Pullman High School and personally coached his wife and two sons. In his prime, he was a respectable distance and middle-distance runner with Olympic aspirations that were cut short by a four-year stint in the Vietnam War. I have no idea how well he ran, whether he was gifted, hardworking or both. He had started to run for Washington State University just before entering the war so nobody, including himself, knew his potential as a runner. Notwithstanding, he was the pied piper of coaches.

Coach Mike understood the challenges and commitment of running at an elite level, although more importantly, he understood the kids. Rather than focusing on medals, places or acclaim, he emphasized personal records or "PRs." Every kid worked for and against themselves. This focus on personal achievement rather than on accolades and awards taught kids the value of trying and of working toward a goal. Not everyone was a winner, only those who tried and nearly everyone did. Mei was immediately receptive and quickly became one of his best young runners. She loved running with the older faster runners, she reveled in being promoted to the competitive group and she bonded with her Mike-appointed personal trainers: collegiate runners from the Washington State University track team.

Three times a week Mike had her running tempo or interval runs, repeated high and very high intensity runs, respectively, that increase an athlete's oxygen carrying capacity and extend their ability to run faster for longer periods of time. I feared, naturally, that the strain and pain could push her away from the sport, one that I realized she had the potential to master. By contrast, Mike taught her not to fear the pain and in a cliché Zen-like fashion to embrace it.

"Distance and middle-distance runners have to learn to run in pain," he said. "If you're not uncomfortable from the very first step, you're not running right." Try teaching *that* to an 8 year old.

Mei sprinted much faster than boys and girls her age as well as most kids two or three years older. She also practiced with endurance athletes almost twice her age. Although I was always athletic, as a child I was small and "wiry" just like she was. I was also faster than most other kids at least until puberty; they got muscular while I stayed wiry. The situation is worse for girls who generally run slower after puberty than before. Indeed, the anatomical changes necessary for female reproduction develop at a cost to other physiological systems and none is good for running fast or far. Fearing Meilani could share my pubertal fate, we had her run a diversity of events including the 100m, 400m and 800m.

Mei dominated all three events for three years, winning primarily first-place medals and an occasional second. Most of these meets were organized by United States of America Track and Field (USATF) or Junior Olympics and thus attracted high-caliber athletes of all ages. She even developed a rival, Natalia, who was a talented young girl from a typical "running family." This fueled many close finishes yet neither girl was ever upset, cried or threw a tantrum. Instead, they hugged and congratulated each other after every race.

An image of their embrace will always be with me. It is an allegory of what I believe is the purest and most beautiful aspect of sport, although its true personal meaning eludes me. I've thought of it many times especially when I see a misbehaving parent or malicious spectator at a youth sporting event. Did they hug from a shared joy of accomplishment, comradery or respect? Sure. Were the hugs scripted? Maybe at some point, but not initially. It really doesn't matter and I never asked Mei why they did it, probably because I didn't want them to stop. I suspect different people would interpret it differently and although I can't pinpoint a specific personal meaning, I recognize, as I'm sure everyone would, its strength in symbolism.

Another image or vision, one that is far less ambiguous also comes to mind often. It's an image of that fateful fall morning when I saw Mei really run for the first time and I asked myself, "Was she really that good?"

I was clearly caught in the moment, hypnotized by a mystic morning and electrifying experience and although I was cognizant of bias, I lacked perspective. This of course is common among parents and especially young parents, but I was a scientist, a professor, an internationally recognized expert in muscle developmental biology who had published research articles in scientific journals exploring muscle strength and the biomechanics of exercise. I even taught a course to honors students instructing techniques for objective reasoning: "Science as a Way of Knowing." I nevertheless questioned, as I still do, whether my emotions were clouding my professional judgment or to the contrary, whether the latter was suppressing a genuine and justified excitement.

It was clear from an early age that Mei ran very, very well. She enjoyed competition and was herself highly competitive. It was also clear that although she wallowed in the social experience of organized play, the act of playing meant more to her than the context of play. Yes, she was gifted and this was crystal clear. What wasn't clear then and now, however, is whether possessing a gift is enough. This of course depends on the definition of "enough," which itself is as amorphic as the *IT* used all too often in defining talent. Indeed, having "enough" of anything is defined by subjective limits that when misunderstood or misapplied can lead to excesses, abuse and even moral misgivings.

MEILANI'S TAKE (15 YEARS OLD)

Sports is an amazing thing. It's more than just play and the sporting experience is more than just fun. Most kids can remember the sound of wind whistling across their ears as they run or the backyard arguments with friends and family that ensue from playing backyard games, but competing in organized events, especially as part of a team, is very different. It can also be very scary and in many ways is an adventure. I've been playing sports my whole life, which I know isn't very long, but my experiences have still taught me a significant amount. One of the most important lessons I've learned is how to handle and even understand loss. I'm not always going to get what I want and sometimes I just have to "deal with it." Complaining never helps and if I'm being honest, it never makes me feel any better. I don't like to lose. In fact, I hate losing, but learning to handle loss in sports will help me cope with losses in life, losses that will no doubt be much more substantial and impactful than losing a challenge on the ball or a race to the finish line.

Even early in my life, I remember being better at sports than most kids my age. I took the practices more seriously and was faster and stronger, despite my tiny size. We lived in Moscow, Idaho, a small rural college town that in no way resembles Moscow, Russia. As with many other small towns, competition and talent were rare and my soccer team barely had enough girls to compete. Our regional league was composed of boys, girls and mixed-sex teams and often combined age groups. I loved playing against the boys, not because I liked the attention but because of the pride I felt when their eyes watered after losing to "just girls." Boys and girls weren't physically different at that age, but boys were raised to be superior to girls in this community and their egos, even at such a young age, were above the clouds. They were also as fragile as eggs. Losing to girls was disgraceful in their minds and the same prepubescent voices that teased us before the game could be heard whining to their mommies afterward. We never lost to a team of boys and we loved it.

Our team was competitive but not great. We beat almost all of the teams in our area and would usually win or tie teams from larger towns and cities. Our coach played soccer in college and she seemed to understand the game better than most of our club's coaches, at least for our age group. She was patient and calm and her practices were always fun. I liked her. I liked learning from her and I liked playing for her yet I didn't like her "coaching." She had a horrible habit of playing favorites and although I was one of her favorites, I like to think that I actually earned my position whereas her daughter did not. Yeah, it's one of *those* situations.

The girl was tall with long blond hair and a wide strong frame, reminiscent of a young Viking warrioress. She had the strongest shot on the team but no accuracy. Even when she concentrated and took her time, it was as if she shot with her eyes closed, shanking the ball in every direction except toward the goal or a teammate. She was never focused during games and would often walk when others ran. I was very young, but I can still feel the seething anger when I remember the Viking sitting down in the middle of the field, in the middle of a game, in many games. My teammates begged from the bench just for a chance to touch the ball while the Viking rested her weary legs watching girls run past up and down the field. It was almost a decade ago and I still get angry thinking about it.

Chapter 2

I loved practice, I loved the games, I loved our coach, but I didn't love the nepotism. Even at a young age, this hung over the team like a black cloud raining jealousy and dissent onto everyone except our coach and the Viking. This was my first competitive team and this experience was my introduction to human nature and the personal imperfections that can sour anything, even playing soccer.

Looking back, I wonder if the coach was trying to help her daughter or herself. Was she playing the Viking to avoid a tantrum or to help the Viking improve? Did she notice the resentment brewing among the girls? Why couldn't she see the obvious, that the Viking stunk and if I'm perfectly honest, usually didn't want to play? I can't fault the coach too much because without her enthusiasm and encouragement, I may have never learned to love the *Beautiful Game*. I may have also been ill prepared to face the challenges of future coaches and teams.

I don't want to misrepresent my feelings about competitive soccer, my personal experiences or team sports in general. The negative experiences were minor by comparison to the positive and in many ways created opportunities to learn. Running track was a similarly positive experience and even more rewarding, although it was also far more difficult. I began running track after a year of playing soccer and joined the Comets, a track club located about 10 miles away in Pullman, Washington, home of Washington State University. Running and track came natural to me and I was immediately successful. My legs never tired and I won almost every race no matter the distance. I even think playing soccer helped with track. It made me more aggressive, more competitive and more willing to fight to the finish.

I was the smallest kid on the Comets. Being tiny may have been a disadvantage in soccer, but it was not in track, at least not in the running events. I loved everything about the sport. I especially loved experimenting with different events and tried sprints, distance, high jump, long jump, anything that caught my interest. There were kids of all ages, from first to 12th grade, but few matched my dedication or competitive spirit. I have always had a strong desire to win and the opportunity to experiment with so many events catered to my lack of focus; there was always so much to do.

The Gift

Our team was led by "Coach Mike" who knew everything about every event and was universally loved. I honestly don't remember anyone ever saying a bad word about Coach Mike.

He took me aside one day and told me that I had something special inside and that he wanted me to work with a private distance coach. She was a student athlete on the Washington State University track team and volunteered to help Coach Mike over the summer. I don't know what she saw in my messy ponytail and crooked teeth, but we immediately bonded. Her workouts were creative and fun and they changed every day: 200 speed repeats, interval ladders, hill repeats or long easy runs. The change took the routine out of the repetition, creating surprise and anxiety, but it was never dull and she always ran with me adding encouragement with every step. I competed in many different events and although I medaled in every race over the first three years, my strength was clearly in distance events. The more I ran the more I realized that track was my sport. It was my calling.

Track meets are always stressful. If you mess up in soccer, no worries, you still have the whole game to make up for it and your teammates always have your back. If you mess up in track, you lose. There is no room for error. I always needed to win and never wanted to disappoint my dad, so before a meet I tried my best to focus. I recited strategy and my splits—target times to designated distances—and I warmed up early. I usually talked to the other girls in the staging area, but as soon as we walked out and the smell of rubber hit my nose, my mind switched to winning. I would match the rhythm of my breathing to the pace of my steps, just like during a race. I thought about all those race pace workouts and how they'd help me hit my splits. After the gun, I'd clear the pack and lock in my pace, remembering to run *through* not *to* the finish line, wondering when the burning in my legs would hit, breathing harder when it did and feeling it dissipate with every breath.

Just as how I would describe the start of a comic book, you should know that I had a nemesis. Her name was Natalia and the only time we saw each other was at large meets. Moscow and Pullman were both small college towns so we almost always traveled to larger cities for competitions, usually Spokane or even Eugene, Oregon. We ran the same events

Chapter 2

and both of our parents thought their child could beat the other. I usually won, but it always came down to the last few steps, except for one fateful time when her foot fell just ahead of mine. I vowed to never let that happen again.

The next time we met was at the United States Track and Field Northwest Regional Championship where she and I were running what became a very memorable 800m race. The stands were full and my heart was beating in my throat. This was the most nervous I had ever felt and despite it being a cool day, Natalia's ginger hair burned red, lighting the track on fire. She was bigger than I was and looked very intimidating. We were the highest-seeded runners in the field and were lined up next to each other with our toes barely nestled behind the white line. Before I had time to think about clearing the field and especially her, the starting gun popped and we both leapt out of the pack.

She immediately pulled ahead of me. I locked in my pace and focused on hitting my marks. On our second and last lap, I narrowed the lead or "reeled her in" to just a few meters, trailing by only two or three steps. We were rounding the third turn and approaching the back straightaway. I could see my dad watching from the 200-meter mark where he'd call out my splits, helping me stay on pace. His voice rang in my ear telling me to kick early since I was behind. My legs burned and throbbed as I moved closer and closer. Her head turned quickly to see where I was. She heard me coming, she felt it. We were quickly approaching the last turn and I knew if I passed now and protected the rail, she would have to pass wide on the turn. I looked inside, but there wasn't enough room so I moved to the edge of lane 2. She sensed my shift and took a step wide toward the second lane. I cussed at her in my head as I burst forward again to the outside; she moved with me and I felt the sole of her shoe against my shin.

I watched in slow motion as she flayed out onto the red track. I tried to jump over her, but my feet hit her and I fell, catching myself with my hand and spinning to my side. I got up and started running back to help her up when I heard my dad yell, "GO, GO, KEEP RUNNING!" He was jumping up and down frantically waving me toward the turn. I turned and started sprinting, never looking back. My goal was to win, to beat Natalia.

I passed the finish line and turned to watch her finish about 10 seconds behind me. I was happy with the victory but felt guilty about the accident and immediately apologized. As you'd expect of two 9 year olds, we hugged it out and laughed about the whole thing. There were no accusations or finger pointing, just two friends caught up in the moment, but as we were walking to the exit an elderly man wearing a large sun hat stormed up to me and began yelling, "You should be ashamed of yourself!" His bony finger waving in front of my nose with every word. I stood there frozen. What do I do? What should I say? Did I really do something wrong? Who is this guy and where's my dad?

I stared at his red face and angry eyes and I can still see that bony finger in my mind. My chest hurt with every word he screamed and each second I stood there my guilt grew and grew. "You cheated! You did it on purpose! You should be disqualified!"

Natalia's mom came running, pushed him to the side and immediately began scolding him. It was her father, Natalia's grandfather, and I guess he got a little too caught up in the race. "Shut up Dad, how dare you! She's just a little girl!" She then turned to me, apologizing, and congratulated me on the win. My eyes were swollen with tears and I remember thinking, "Don't cry, you did nothing wrong."

I often think about that day, the bony finger and his red-hot face. Maybe my dad should have just told me to help her up. Maybe I should have passed wider. Who knows? What I do know is that I didn't deserve to be berated by a strange old man in front of all those people. I also know that despite our age and competitiveness, neither Natalia nor I wanted the incident to ruin our friendship, which was really an acquaintanceship or even a friendly rivalry. Why were two children able to solve something an adult couldn't? Why were we the proverbial adults in the room? As I walked back to my dad's car, I remember feeling confused and couldn't stop thinking about the race and that angry old man. Something I didn't realize in that sunlit parking lot, with my small hand clutched in the protection of my father's, was that this experience was only the beginning. There would be many bad parents and even a few bad coaches in my future.

The true value of sports is learning how to win, how to lose, how to work as a team and, most importantly, how to challenge yourself. It teaches the difference between *not getting your way* and *not getting your opportunity* and how to live with both outcomes. It's okay to get upset when a child athlete loses, makes mistakes or when things just don't go their way, but adults must always—I can't believe I have to say this—remember to act like adults. After all, a child athlete's goal is to have fun. Period. We're not thinking about scholarships or championships, at least not in the beginning. We just want to have fun.

CHAPTER 3

Body and Mind

Life isn't binary. Contemporary media might argue otherwise in relentlessly pitting X versus Y, Republican versus Democrat, blue collar versus white collar, rich versus poor, *et cetera*. Yet the true reality of life is that everything, literally everything is nuanced.

Health, for example, is often discussed from a physiological or mental perspective with mutual exclusivity, that one doesn't necessarily affect the other, that fitness, like sanity, is somehow tissue specific. The American healthcare system in particular exacerbates this false dichotomy with different regulations governing access and reimbursement to medical and psychological services. Providers for these respective services rarely work in the same clinic and almost always collaborate via referral or consultation rather than in co-managed care. Exceptions are reserved for the unique, severe or rare, ignoring a well-documented shortcoming in access to mental health services for everyone except the privileged. The problem is even reflected in the terminology itself as "medical" and "psychological" are presumed distinct as if mental health is somehow distinguished from medical or at best is a sub-field.

Academia echoes a similar false dichotomy by pitting intellectual and athletic development in a zero-sum game. Schools rarely excel at both and are particularly scrutinized if success is (a) disparate and (b) conflicts with regional politics. We previously lived in Idaho where a small conservative community eliminated advanced placement courses from their high school curriculum to preserve the status of their football program. The sport wasn't to be eliminated but would have received less funding and despite the extremely low likelihood that any of the players from this tiny town could compete for a university scholarship, regardless of division, the parents and politicians almost universally supported the change. Likewise, our current district in Maryland, which is textbook progressive (pardon the pun), regularly underfunds their athletic programs and to be perfectly honest, they're embarrassingly bad. The pathetic nature of these programs extends throughout the district and has, I suspect, contributed to the growth of an extremely lucrative club sports market that primarily caters to the wealthy.

One could argue that the overemphasis of organized sports at all levels of academia not only distracts but also detracts as funds and fundraising disproportionately support sports at the expense of academics, which ironically brings us full circle to the problem of binary. Why do we accept these false dichotomies? Why do we prioritize academic and athletic development at the expense of one another? Why, as a culture, do we presume that the development of our children's physical and mental health is mutually exclusive when in fact the functional status of neural and non-neural tissues is inextricably linked? Indeed, changes in mental health are almost always accompanied by changes in physical health while the converse is also true.

Several studies have explored this relationship in detail and although the physiological benefits of exercise are well known, often repeated in mantra fashion and foundational to the health and fitness industries, the public's understanding of mental health benefits are anecdotal at best and most often misunderstood. This is especially true for children.

Many academic research studies have established links between physical activity and cognition as well as with academic achievement. More mechanistic studies have established "cause-and-effect" relationships with controlled studies and even with animals. Indeed, the neuroscience world has extensively explored the effects of physical activity, exercise and environmental enrichment on the cognitive abilities of laboratory animals down to the molecular level. Published reviews regularly summarize large bodies of work, assessing rigor and presenting novel experimental paradigms and models to be tested, all of which fuels more growth in the field.

The question isn't whether exercise enriches cognition, as this is extremely well established, but how and I mean specifically *how* does this occur? What genes are involved? What biochemical pathways are activated or suppressed? What neurological processes are involved and can they be manipulated to improve treatment outcomes for neurological diseases? The answer to this last question you'll be happy to learn is an emphatic YES!

"Physical activity" in these studies is generally defined as any muscle-inspired bodily movement that comes with an energetic cost, meaning that nutrients are consumed and metabolic byproducts are produced. This is important because the byproducts can be quantified directly in bodily fluids or in muscle biopsies. They can also be indirectly measured in real time while animals or human subjects are exercising, as with respiration and calorimetry. This enables researchers to gauge intensity and to normalize activity, ensuring apples-to-apples comparisons. Such invasive tools are generally reserved for controlled laboratory studies whereas population-based studies use surveys and complex statistics, all advanced tools of the experimental exercise physiologist.

It is important to understand that within a scientific context, this and other seemingly familiar terms have highly specific definitions that may differ from the non-scientific. Physical activity and "exercise," for example, are not interchangeable as the latter is a subset of the former. Exercise is always highly structured and its goal is to improve "physical fitness," which is a physiological state that can be quantified and assessed scientifically. Exercises are often tailored to achieve a specific fitness goal like increasing strength, endurance or flexibility; preventing injury; improving athletic performance or reducing disease risk factors. "Fitness" is exclusively used in these studies to define physiological functions as mental or psychological functions are defined as "cognition." This term encompasses a variety of intellectual functions including memory, perception, attention, reasoning and problem solving, to name a few, and is itself an entirely unique field of science. Some studies examine "learning" or the gain of new knowledge through cognitive processes and either directly test subjects or simply monitor metrics of learned behavior. In animals, this could involve navigating a maze or performing reward-based tasks, while studies of students usually assess academic achievement by monitoring performance on standardized exams.

Animals are generally used to explore the underlying mechanisms of physical activity on cognitive functions or learning. These studies often examine or even manipulate gene function, neurogenesis (formation of new neurons), synapse formation (connections between neurons) and/or neural activity (electrical firing of neurons), and although mice are the most common model, the cognitive benefit of enhanced physical activity has been demonstrated in a variety of vertebrate species. A favorite and recent example is a study performed at the University of Guelph using the amphibious, hermaphroditic, self-fertilizing and skin-breathing killifish *Kryptolebias marmoratus*, a mangrove fish that frequently crawls on land to find prey and avoid predation.[1] Seriously cool!

Not only did repeated terrestrial exercise or exposure to land improve spatial learning, which was tested using a "bifurcating T-maze" where fish learn to navigate obstacles in a single-point two-choice (left- versus right-turn) maze, it also increased the number of proliferating cells in a brain region important for spatial cognition, the dorsolateral pallium. Previous studies by the same group of scientists, led by Dr. Patricia Wright, determined that terrestrial exercise increases muscle mass and aerobic capacity while simultaneously increasing jumping distance and time to exhaustion.

These results are far from trivial and in fact have meaning well beyond the mangroves. Exercise, however unique to the system being tested, literally changed the structure and function of muscle, all as expected. In addition, it also changed the structure and function of the brain and in a region important for the learning task being performed, which should excite everyone's inner nerd. This particular physical activity involved muscle contractions, stress responses, sensory excitation, metabolite utilization, enhanced cognition and activation of countless other physiological systems known to influence or be influenced by the brain, and although it's impossible to identify a single key factor responsible and difficult to prioritize the relevant physiological influences, the study proves a very salient point: exercise affects neurological change.

Thousands of other studies with more conventional animal models, like mice and rats, belabor this point and have even identified the underlying genes, biochemical pathways and neurological systems involved and as with the killifish, neurogenesis and synaptic plasticity are enhanced, particularly with endurance exercise. Neuroscientists and ethologists have further explored the structure-function relationship of such changes in animal and human subjects and have determined that exercise-induced cognitive improvement occurs through changes in "episodic memory," defined as obtaining, storing and recalling information (aka learning), and from "long-term potentiation," which is the formation of neural connections required for learning and memory. Exercise even functions as a therapeutic for many neurological diseases and is arguably the leading lifestyle intervention for improving cognition in stroke, dementia, Alzheimer's and Parkinson's patients. It is also very well known to delay normal age-related cognitive decline.

The myriad physiological systems recruited with physical activity, especially with strenuous exercise, are directly or indirectly connected to the brain. This can involve electrical signals from sensory nerves that connect peripheral tissues like muscle and the heart to the central nervous system (i.e., brain and spinal cord). It additionally involves chemical signals secreted into blood or into spaces outside of tissues. Examples include hormones or, in the case of muscle, myokines, which are hormone-like chemicals secreted by muscles. Myokines regulate fat and bone in addition to muscle and have also been shown to cross the "blood-brain barrier," an evolutionary conserved structure that functions like a building's concrete foundation and prevents exposure to foreign pathogens and other hostile factors. Chemicals that cross this barrier under normal healthy conditions are meant to be there and for one particular myokine, irisin, its purpose is to regulate neural development. Spoiler alert, irisin release is stimulated with exercise!

Irisin is derived from a large protein called "fibronectin-domain III containing 5"—initiate obligatory eye roll now. This protein is abbreviated as FNDC5 and is bound to the outermost membranes of skeletal and cardiac muscle cells. It is also produced by the intracranial arteries that feed the brain and to a much lesser degree by some neurons. A small part of FNDC5 is found inside the cell, another is embedded within the outer lipid membrane of the cell, while the majority of the protein extends outside the cell. Each of these regions or domains serve a distinct purpose and although the function of the intracellular domain remains elusive, the extracellular domain is the most functionally relevant to exercise and is the source of irisin.

Consider an analogy where FNDC5 is an "irisin bank" tethered to the muscle cell membrane. Exercise makes a withdrawal using a protease debit card, an enzyme that literally cuts the extracellular domain of FNDC5 into two separate parts: a small piece with no known function and a much larger chuck, irisin. The liberated pieces are then free to move about the space between the muscle cell membrane and blood vessels or to enter the bloodstream where irisin is carried throughout the body.

Hormones and myokines like irisin are considered chemical messengers that help different cells and tissues communicate across often great distances. From a molecular perspective, a hormone traversing the circulatory system is akin to the space shuttle galivanting around the solar system. Messengers aren't directed *per se* to a particular location, like a letter to a mailbox, but move randomly from one extracellular or tissue compartment to another. Their fate is ultimately determined by interactions with other molecules or groups of molecules that in turn determine where and how the messengers act. Unlike the nervous system that communicates via pinpointed electric signals, hardwired from regulator (e.g., brain) to effector (e.g., muscle), chemical messaging functions like a dip net extending into a current of migrating fish. Some fish are too large for the net, some swim between the eyes while others fit just right. Netting of fish in this analogy represents the chemical messenger binding to a receptor that then triggers a cascade of enzymatic reactions to change cellular and tissue behaviors. The type and number of receptors differ between tissues, which explains why only select tissues are affected by a given messenger. Tissue growth, embryological development, cardiac and renal function, in fact every aspect of every physiological system is controlled by chemical messengers and this includes a muscle-to-brain interaction.

A relatively recent study published in the journal *Nature Metabolism* perfectly illustrates the importance of this interaction, at least from a biomedical perspective.[2] It may also explain how exercise in general improves cognition in a variety of vertebrate species, possibly even our favorite killifish. A Harvard medical group led by Dr. Christiane Wrann used genetic engineering to remove the FNDC5 gene from mice and eliminate the source of irisin. These FNDC5 "knockout" mice were then included in exercise experiments that assessed the impact of running on age-related cognitive decline. Irisin's role in the muscle-to-brain interaction was also studied in mouse models of Parkinson's disease.

Mice love to run and will even compete for access to running wheels, which are often used to study the effects of exercise on myriad different physiological and behavioral systems. Mice that run perform much better than sedentary mice in spatial learning tests as, for example, the time required to navigate a complex maze. They also outperform sedentary mice in the Morris water maze, a swimming test where mice are challenged to find and, more importantly, remember the location of a platform sunken in a pool of murky water. Cognitive improvement with exercise occurs in mice of all ages and results not from an enriched environment *per se* as this has been extensively tested but specifically from running.

Dr. Wrann's group used the water maze test to determine if irisin knockout mice—those literally lacking the FNDC5 gene that contains irisin—could still benefit from exercise. Before starting the experiment, however, scientists first performed a battery of tests and confirmed that knockout mice lacked motor impairments and were athletically equivalent but not superior to normal or "wild-type" mice. They then divided knockout and wild-type mice into separate testing groups. Sedentary mice could freely move about their cage while the exercised mice were provided access to running wheels.

Over the period of six days, exercised wild-type mice clearly outperformed sedentary wild-type mice in daily water maze tests. This confirmed hundreds of previous studies reporting the cognitive benefit of exercise and served as the scientists' positive control. By contrast, exercise had no effect on the knockout mice, suggesting that the cognitive benefits of running require FNDC5 and irisin. The short six-day testing period is highly significant as this duration is too short to provide any athletic benefit and even if it did, the effect would be equal in both wild-type and knockout mice as both groups ran the same amount.

Pattern separation tests, those testing the ability to remember negative reinforcement in the form of a minor but irritating electric shock, were then used to determine if cognitive improvement was limited to spatial recognition or if other learning tasks improved. As before, exercise had no effect on the knockout mice while it enhanced performance in the wild-type mice. Anxiety- and depression-like behavior was then assessed in knockout mice to determine if they lacked motivation, but their behavior was normal. The only detected deficit was in the ability of exercise to enhance cognition.

The study's *pièce de résistance* came when scientists used a gene therapeutic to restore irisin and in turn the cognitive benefits of exercise. The treatment also altered structures in the brain important to cognition and was later demonstrated to partially prevent neurodegeneration in a mouse model of Alzheimer's disease. Although these particular results are unrelated to the topic of exercise, they are far more important and are being used to develop a novel clinical treatment for this and other neurodegenerative diseases, possibly Parkinson's.

FNDC5 and irisin are pieces of the exercise-induced cognitive improvement puzzle; pretty important pieces, but pieces nonetheless. Indeed, there's little evidence to suggest that irisin alone is entirely responsible for all of the cognitive benefits originating from exercise. Even if one subscribes to such molecular reductionism, you couldn't ignore the receptors and intracellular responses that mediate irisin's actions or the different neurological responses or the metabolites fueling the brain and muscle or myriad other physiological processes capable of potentiating irisin's influences. Irisin isn't the holy grail of exercise physiology. It is, however, a *mechanism of action* linking muscle activity and exercise to the neural plasticity that causes cognitive improvement, and this in turn explains how physical activity can be so strongly associated with high-order and complex cognitive outcomes like academic achievement.

An exercised-induced rise in blood irisin levels also occurs in people, especially with endurance exercise, while the myokine has additionally been identified in our brains. This suggests that people and possibly all mammals if not all vertebrates, including killifish, can benefit from the neurotropic and cognition-enhancing actions of exercise-induced irisin release. Such findings are far from surprising and although only a few irisin studies have been performed with human subjects, the field is poised to explode. This is largely due to its therapeutic potential in treating the neurological diseases noted earlier but also because it explains the well-known cognitive benefits that occur with physical activity even in children and adolescents.

The positive and causative link between exercise and cognition is admittedly much more established in adults than it is in children of any age. This can also be said for most biomedical phenomena as children are rarely subjects of clinical trials outside pediatric-specific diseases and have similarly low representation in basic clinical studies. Epidemiologists and behavior psychologists have nevertheless conducted dozens of studies with children as young as 4 years old and with a variety of physical activities and sports. Outcome measures from early cognitive development in the very young to academic achievement in teenagers have been assessed while a variety of cognitive (e.g., changes to working memory, language skills, attention span, etc.) and physiological (e.g., brain structure, neural activity) mechanisms have been explored and even correlated to the outcomes.

From a cognitive perspective, acute physical activity has been consistently demonstrated to improve the time required to perform a mental task or "processing speed." It not only helps you think quicker but also increases attention span and improves skills required for multi-tasking referred to as "cognitive flexibility" or the ability to rapidly and accurately refocus thinking. Chronic bouts of physical activity have similar effects and additionally improve working or short-term memory and possibly even language skills. These basic cognitive benefits have even been linked to academic achievement.

Chapter 3

Dr. Joseph Donnelly, an exercise physiologist at the University of Kansas Medical Center, and Dr. Charles Hillman, an exercise psychologist now at Northeastern University, led a team of scientists in a meta-analysis of 64 studies that interrogated the impact of physical activity and fitness on cognition and learning.[3] Meta-analyses are extremely informative and help clarify confusion that often arises from apple-to-orange comparisons between studies. They also incorporate highly rigorous statistical tests while qualitatively assessing the rigor of the studies themselves.

The meta-analysis further assessed studies of brain structure, using magnetic resonance imaging (MRI), and brain function, using electroencephalography (EEG) or functional MRI. The team additionally analyzed 73 separate studies to determine if physical activity and sports programs influence performance on standardized achievement tests or concentration/attention. The children's ages ranged from 5 to 13 in these studies and some participated in controlled laboratory tests. The others were part of cross-sectional longitudinal studies where data from large student populations were collected at a particular time.

This meta-analysis epitomizes the field and serves as a wonderful example for conducting and controlling such analyses. Eligibility criteria for finding and selecting studies were strictly enforced and each of the selected studies were assessed for quality and bias. This prevents poorly designed studies, for example, those with very small number of participants, those with participants from only high- or low-achieving schools or those that simply used bad math, from affecting the overall conclusions. Their approach was highly thorough and their conclusions are justified and carefully worded, free from hyperbole. The authors were not out to sell but to educate. They also did their best to simplify comparisons, following the law of parsimony, which is less elegantly known as the "keep it simple stupid" or KISS principle, by asking just two fundamental questions:

1. Do physical activity and aerobic fitness influence cognition and learning as well as brain structure and function?
2. Do physical activity, aerobic fitness and physical education influence academic achievement?

Answering the first question was a relatively easy task. It relied more heavily on outcomes like memory or perception that can be easily quantified without producing large amounts of variability. Conclusions were also consistently confirmed between studies even when different cognition or learning outcomes were measured. Indeed, the underlying hypothesis was overwhelmingly confirmed: physical activity and aerobic fitness had a positive effect on cognition, learning and the brain. Even single bouts of physical activity were effective while the brain structures that increased in size or activity coincided with regions well known to support complex cognitive processes.

Although a limited number of controlled studies were included in the assessment, data from these studies again reflected a positive relationship. This suggests that increased physical activity/fitness not only *correlates* to improved cognition/learning but actually *causes* it. Greater amounts of physical activity or performing the activities at higher intensities were further demonstrated to produce more substantial effects. "Just do it" clearly works while "do it with intensity" works even better!

Answering the second question proved more difficult yet was in some ways even more informative. Academic achievement on standardized tests was primarily used as the outcome measure and although the overall results were mixed, they were not completely inconclusive. Cross-sectional and longitudinal studies demonstrated a general positive effect on academic achievement. Controlled studies with a limited number of participants, however, produced mixed results. Some revealed positive associations whereas others revealed no or even negative effects. Physical activity would be demonstrated to influence math, for example, but not reading or to improve achievement in boys but not girls or *vice versa*.

These results, in hindsight, were not unexpected as it's often difficult and sometimes impossible to completely control for effort or aptitude in behavioral studies, and this difficulty is exacerbated when using a small number of participants. This appeared to be the case with many physical education studies as attempts to increase physical activity—the thing hypothesized to improve academic achievement—failed.

By contrast, studies where physical activity was directed with coaching consistently demonstrated a positive effect on academic achievement.

Study groups were also controlled in these studies to avoid selection bias, which in this case could have placed a bunch of geniuses in one group and a bunch of college administrators or politicians, the polar opposite of geniuses, in the other.

Authors of the Donnelly/Hillman meta-analysis were careful to not overstate their conclusions and even described the overall effect of physical education on academic achievement as "neutral." Several other studies including meta-analyses have been published since the Donnelly/Hillman study, providing additional evidence supporting a positive effect of physical activity on various cognitive functions. Not to beat a dead horse, but cognitive functions like processing speed, attention, working memory, flexibility and language learning have all been demonstrated to improve with physical activity in healthy children and with some studies in children with documented learning disorders like attention-deficit/hyperactivity disorder.

This latter effect is reminiscent of studies performed in animal models of neurodegeneration and in human stroke, dementia, Alzheimer's and Parkinson's patients. Indeed, physical activity is far more than a means to maintain a healthy body and mind; it is also a therapy. In obese children with or without type 2 diabetes mellitus, which is arguably the most significant pediatric public health problem of our time, physical activity improves blood glucose regulation by similarly improving insulin sensitivity and as a result, the overall metabolic profile. It also strengthens bones and improves cardiorespiratory fitness and can lower mortality risk in children with type 1 diabetes mellitus, which unlike type 2 can be fatal if poorly controlled.

The medical benefits of physical activity in children are literally too numerous to list, that is unless we revisit that dead horse. Asthma; cardiovascular disease; risks for developing breast, skin and other cancers; muscular dystrophies; et cetera, et cetera, *et cetera* can all be addressed in part with some form of physical activity. This is likely as true for children as it is for adults, although the evidence is not nearly as well established, yet it's still very convincing. Physical activity can even prevent development of mental health problems in adolescence, which according to the Centers for Disease Control and Prevention, the World Health Organization, UNICEF and literally every scientific agency that monitors and studies pediatric mental health is a serious and mostly untreated problem that appears to be worsening.

All of these studies—those with healthy adults, with the elderly and those with neurodegenerative diseases, with children of various ages in controlled or cross-sectional studies, with children from economically depressed communities and those with metabolic or mental disorders or with serious and eventually fatal neuromuscular diseases, even studies performed with mice and fish—all of these studies provide tangible evidence of the "body and mind" relationship. They indicate beyond a shadow of a doubt that physical and mental health are not only inseparable but that one can be used to develop and improve the other.

Eliminating stress, for example, is well known to improve athletic performance at all levels of play and is probably crucial to a healthy youth sporting experience. Professional athletes and coaches as well as sports psychologists commonly use repetitive practice, visualization, meditation, yoga, music, routines bordering on obsessive-compulsive disorder and even hypnosis to de-stress their athletes, which really makes one wonder why youth coaches scream all the time. Seriously, why?

Stress feeds competitive or sport-related performance anxiety and eventually burnout. These are two of the most common and long-term threats to young competitive athletes and the causes are myriad. Both can and do result from abusive coaching but also from parental and self-imposed pressures, poor team dynamics, malicious spectators and a host of other dysfunctionalities. There really is no causal consensus, which for obvious reasons shouldn't be surprising. Each person, athlete and experience is different and what may be debilitating to some is a common shrug-off to others. Reception does not equate to perception.

Early sport specialization is a common investigational theme among academics studying child sports psychology. It's also, in my personal and professional opinion, a strawman argument. The term itself lacks a consensus definition and many studies rely upon self-reporting or anecdotal evidence, which is notoriously unreliable. Very few studies report long-term psychological outcomes and those that do qualify their conclusions with disqualifying words like "potential," "might" and "possibly." The theme itself is in many ways the excuse *du jour*, albeit for good reason.

CHAPTER 3

Doing too much of any one thing gets boring. This is hardly a Nobel Prize–winning discovery, but it does explain how early specialization—emphasis on *early*—potentially contributes to competitive anxiety and burnout. These aren't mutually exclusive problems, mind you, as anxiety is commonly cited as a motivation for burnout. Both problems also occur among collegiate athletes and adults that are years if not decades beyond specialization and who have either habituated to a sport's unique eccentricities or have openly embraced them. Thus, it's difficult to accept that specialization *per se* is the root cause for anxiety and burnout rather than one of many contributing factors.

Overcoming anxiety is an adolescent rite of passage and although young athletes and non-athletes experience anxiety at similar rates, anxiety and burnout occur at higher rates in young versus adult athletes. Rates are also higher in girls than boys.

Several attempts to alleviate anxiety, to de-stress athletes, have been tested in the field. Some studies were controlled, some weren't and nearly all reported beneficial reductions in perceived stress and, for those that measured it, improved athletic performance. This is all highly encouraging, although the skeptic in me inherently distrusts anything that's so universally successful.

I don't question whether mental training with interventions like mindfulness, psychological skills training or cognitive behavioral therapy can effectively de-stress an athlete or that alleviating anxiety can enhance athletic performance and prevent burnout. This is all very well established. I do, however, question whether some of the numerous and diverse interventions tested could broadly function as a specific cure-all solution when each requires some level of personalization. Meditating to music, for example, won't work with people who don't like music or who associate it with trauma or loss. What does work and what appears common if not foundational to all of the successful interventions is (1) changing the competitive environment from negative reinforcement to personal achievement and (2) "focusing on the now."

The much-maligned negative reinforcement is in fact a necessary component of any teaching environment as, for example, with grade scales: low grades reinforce via negativity, high grades via positivity. The system works because it's balanced and regulated with both positive and negative reinforcements on the same scale. Teachers manipulate the scale with curves and extra credit, skewing it toward positivity, while bad grades signal teachers, staff and parents to intervene. Negative reinforcement is not inherently malicious, at least not when properly used, but imagine a classroom skewed the other way. Where negativity dominates, where teachers constantly scream at students and rarely if ever praise or reward their efforts. Would your child enjoy learning this way? Would learning excite them or fill them with anxiety? Would they excel or quit?

The originator of mindfulness-based stress reduction or simply "mindfulness," Dr. Jon Kabat-Zinn, PhD, is a retired professor of medicine at the University of Massachusetts. He founded the Center for Mindfulness in 1971 and treated patients with stress-related disease for over 40 years. Mindfulness is defined as "paying attention in a particular way: on purpose, in the present moment, and nonjudgmentally" and has been used with great fanfare to treat patients, soldiers, business executives, healthcare providers, many other professional disciplines and, yes, athletes of all ages. If it can reduce medical errors, improve surgical performance and keep doctors and nurses in the clinic, saving lives instead of sinking putts, it can likely help your child score a goal or basket without quitting the team or the classroom.

Mindfulness is a structured form of meditation. It differs from psychological skills training or cognitive behavioral therapy that teach athletes to alter their feelings or emotional responses to a stressor or stressful situation. Common examples of skills training include setting goals or envisioning situations whereas cognitive behavioral therapy explores the association between thoughts, feelings and behavioral responses. "Focus on the positive" could be an appropriate mantra for either. Mindfulness, by contrast, teaches athletes to focus on everything in the experience, the positive and negative as well as the mundane.

Mindfulness programs are quick to learn and can be integrated into a training plan far more easily and affordably than most other mental training interventions that require a licensed psychologist or psychiatrist. The internet is littered with such programs, many of which are designed for specific sports and age groups, although almost none is backed by a licensed program and most are in my mind suspect. By contrast, affordable mindfulness programs are offered online by the UMass Memorial Medical Center and the Center for Mindfulness.[4]

Classes are available for individuals or groups/teams and are offered as three-day retreats or for weeks-long training programs. Both options could prove difficult financially or logistically for most youth teams but possibly not for entire organizations, clubs or schools. Coaches could also take the classes themselves or even become licensed and then design programs unique to their own team challenges. Typical interventions include exercises in breathing, self-monitoring and "body scanning," which is form of meditation that progressively focuses attention to different body parts. Athletes are taught team values and learn how to assess, act and control value-driven behavior while coaches learn methods to increase engagement and ultimately acceptance of the program. It's not as tree hugging and tofu as you might suspect and it works, not only in sports but in most aspects of people's lives.

I've studied stress for much of my career, how it adversely affects many different physiological systems and tissues, how muscle mass, motor control, cognition, nutrient utilization and storage as well as the immune and digestive systems are all directly influenced by stress hormones. Good mental health is a prerequisite to good physical health and as a corollary, eliminating stress from the competitive environment will undoubtedly improve the athlete and the athletic performance. The converse is also true as both aerobic and resistance training is often used as a therapeutic coping mechanism for chronic and acute stress, especially with clinical depression, anxiety and even post-traumatic stress disorder.

There's little doubt that athletes can benefit from mental training in general or specifically from mindfulness. It should be noted, however, that very few studies were performed with young or even adolescent athletes and although this alone riles the skeptic in me, I'm perfectly comfortable advocating simple algebraic logic. If stress equals anxiety and anxiety produces burnout, then alleviating stress prevents burnout, a well-proven theorem. Anything capable of doing this, therefore, whether it's professional intervention in the form of mental training, meditation or occasional vacations from competition, should always be encouraged.

Most importantly, and this can't be emphasized enough, coaches and parents should always look to eliminate external stressors from the playing experience and to never introduce them. Competition is by definition stressful enough and whether it occurs on a field or in a classroom, over a chessboard or in a boardroom, it compromises emotional states, executive function and athletic or professional performance. Success in such environments is achieved largely by overcoming stress as well as its source, which should be the competition itself or the competitor. It should never be your own coaches, parents or teammates.

My own personal anecdotal experiences as a life-long amateur wannabe athlete with an impeccable record of poor finishes, non-qualifications and humiliating lack of accolades are worth noting even if my winnings or lack thereof are not. I run. I run not for glory or even competition but for myself. I run for my sanity. I run to feel good and look good and to think and do good. My best thoughts about work or life *always* come when I'm running. I run to solve problems. I run to celebrate or commiserate. I run to beat Bob and Puck and Chris and sometimes Alex, actually never Alex, yet I still run. I've run marathons in sweltering heat. I've run near marathons in blizzards, with frozen stalactites hanging from my cap, from my eyelashes and beard, with fingers and toes and ears all numb. I ran the day my father died, weeping with every step. I ran when my mother died yet I can't remember a single step, only my thoughts. My mind and my body are healthy and strong because I run and I want this for my children as much as I want it for myself. A healthy body and a healthy mind. Body *and* mind, one of the same, inseparable.

MEILANI'S TAKE (16 YEARS OLD)
I've heard it a million times, "body and mind, body and mind."

I didn't always grasp the deeper meaning and naively thought of the obvious or literal meaning like "running is good for your health" without seriously considering what a healthy mind was. When I was younger, I thought that playing sports and exercising somehow make you smarter. Pretty silly, right? Maybe not. I now understand the importance of being balanced and how exercise makes my body strong and my mind even stronger, although to be honest, I'm just now learning what this means.

Chapter 3

I've played soccer and run track my whole life and to a certain extent both have helped define who I am, mentally and physically. My personality, my attitude, my competitiveness and drive, my figure, my beauty, my strength and speed are all products of play. I've always been tiny but very athletic and my fondest memories have always involved sports. Dominating kickball in the third grade, being the only girl who could pass the rope climbing challenge in PE class, beating boys on the soccer field and lapping older girls on the track are among my fondest memories. They are also sources of pride and thinking about them fills me with confidence. Being so active also sculpted my body and although I was initially naïve to the effects, I can in no way say that I am unhappy with the outcome or with the healthy appetite that feeds it.

The more I run and harder I practice, the more I eat. Sometimes it's actually hard eating enough and I almost never gain weight. This is a gift in many ways because I never worry about developing a belly or love handles. My appetite is a source of entertainment to my friends who joke about how I'm always snacking, although not always on healthy food. They tend to order balanced meals at restaurants, but I avoid vegetables at all costs. They ask for water; I demand whole milk. They opt out of dessert; I order crème brûlée or brownies à la mode or whatever my heart desires. My dad scolds me for not eating healthy enough and lectures me on the importance of a balanced diet, but I honestly never feel the need to grab an apple instead of a cookie and when I'm most active, I can't get enough cookies.

This gift is also in many ways a curse. Most people worry about being overweight whereas I have the exact opposite concern. No matter how much I eat, I can't gain weight. When I was going through puberty I worried more about my body not changing, if you know what I mean, than how it was changing and I still worry about my ribs showing or how some shirts make me look "flat." When I tell my friends about how I hate missing my periods, they say something like, "You're soooooo lucky, I wish I never had my period." I guess I understand why they look at me as fortunate, but not having a period makes me feel broken. I don't look like my mom when she was my age and I don't look like my friends. There was even a time when I thought my body would never change.

My father told me about a psychological study where boys and girls were questioned about their body image. I was surprised to learn that boys were just as worried as girls about how others viewed them. Sure, I worry, but not like some of my friends who suffer from eating disorders like anorexia or bulimia. I'm not saying I've never skipped a meal because I thought I looked bloated or sucked in my stomach and I completely sympathize with their emotional state because we've all felt insecure at times, but the idea that poor body image could cause someone to torture themselves dumbfounds me. I'm thin because I play, but I'm also strong, healthy and confident. When I'm feeling insecure, I think I look like a cereal box, a door, a table or, if you really want to get creative, a college-ruled crisp sheet of paper. I have no chest, hips, or curves in general, so finding clothes that fit can be very difficult. I avoid things that highlight my insecurities like V necks, which are wasted on me. Shopping for jeans is an "exploration of frustration" because my thighs are disproportionately much bigger than my waist so nothing fits. Until recently, I would never wear a crop top because my ribs would show and I looked sickly. My father says I'm beautiful, but what daughter can trust her dad? They're programmed to say we look amazing. I know this for a fact because he's said I look good in orange and I most definitely do not, if you're wondering.

I think of myself as an optimist and I'm pretty sure my peers do as well. I don't wake up on the wrong side of the bed and only a few of my very close friends have seen me cry. I try to appreciate what I have rather than what I don't and when I feel sad, I compare my worries to what's really worthy of tears, problems my friends are having or something horrible in the news. So what if I'm skinny? So what if I'm flat? So what? I can run fast and I'm healthy. My legs are long, miniskirts are never too short and heels are the biggest form of flattery. I have worked hard for the body I have and I'm proud of it; every muscle, every bony protrusion, every scar represents who I've become. I'm not sure if sports gave me the attitude I have today, but I do know that running, sweating, fighting, yelling and pushing myself have given me my confidence.

When I look into the mirror, I see "thin," not "skinny." There's a difference. Skinny people tumble away in a strong wind, thin people knife through it. Weighing only 110 pounds and standing 5 feet 7 inches tall, nobody would ever describe me as foreboding, yet I'm a lot stronger than I look and my high school soccer coach says I play "twice my size." I made the varsity team as a freshman, eventually starting at left or right wing. The COVID-19 pandemic had shortened our season and all the girls were clamoring for playing time. They also "upped their game" during practice, playing more physical, fouling hard and often. Upperclassmen weren't happy being replaced by a freshman but quickly learned that I can give as well as I receive. I wasn't always a physical player and to be honest, I was kind of a wimp. This all changed when I was 11 and joined the Coyotes, a private club soccer team in Maryland.

The Coyotes were very competitive, very successful and very, very aggressive. We were not only the best team in the state but one of the best in the country and were ranked fourth at one point in time. Our coaches encouraged dirty fouls and extreme aggression. I still laugh when I remember one telling me to dig my fingernails into an opponent's arm. Players were expected to practice how they play, which meant playing hard all the time, never giving up and winning every challenge. When I tried out for the team, I was elbowed in the ribs, knocked to the ground, shoved from behind and practically stripped by the team's official bully who wouldn't stop grabbing my shirt or kicking my feet as I ran. I played scared for months until finally learning to fight back, sometimes harder and in my own creative way. Anticipate the elbows, clamp down on their arms. Bend your knees and lean, step and push into a hit. If they grab your shirt, you grab their shorts; humiliation is a powerful defense.

Was this morally okay? Were the girls able to form real friendships? Do I think this was a healthy environment? No, no and hell no! Was it fun? Yes and no, but that's not the point, at least not yet. Playing on the Coyotes toughened me up mentally and physically and made me a stronger and better player. The experience helped me learn how to deal with bullies and difficult people, to intimidate someone twice my size and, most importantly, to stand up for myself. When I'm older, whether I'm in college, working or just walking down the street, I know I'll meet difficult people. I know there will be bullies in my life. However, I also know how to fight for my rights, how to help a friend in an abusive relationship or how to recover from a breakup. I found my strength years ago, on a soccer field, and I will never lose it.

From an emotional perspective, running is very different from soccer or any other sport. My dad describes it as his "church." I didn't really understand what he meant until I experienced my own religious epiphany of sorts. I usually run in pseudo-rural neighborhoods or along the towpath of the Chesapeake and Ohio or "C&O" Canal, which parallels much of the Potomac River. Exploring new neighborhoods and trying different roads just to see where they lead is always fun and at the same time a little scary. I was on a simple shakeout run, which is an easy recovery run after a hard workout the previous day, and decided to explore a new road that I had always avoided. It was dark and canopied by trees with a very ominous feel. I'm weirdly obsessed with mystery novels and couldn't shake the feeling that I was about to get murdered by someone jumping out from the trees and bushes lining the narrow road. I nervously picked up the pace and as soon as I hit the darkest part of the road where trees seemed to completely shut out all the sunlight, it started to rain. Were the trees crying or warning me? Murder scenes from every mystery novel on my shelf were streaming through my mind. I imagined seeing a body being buried or a scary clown, which was a real craze in our part of the country, grown men dressing up as clowns and walking through the woods. Seriously guys, get a life already.

I remembered seeing a video of a deer slamming into a cross-country runner and somehow convinced myself that deer were out to get me. My pace picked up as all these silly scenarios played in my head until I saw a small red speck hiding past the green haze of leaves. I stopped running and for several minutes sat and stared at a fox tucked away in a small clearing behind the brush. Then came the deer, like an old Disney cartoon, and I stopped caring about the rain or the dark trees or murderous clowns or even my tired legs. I suddenly noticed the faint chirping of birds and the soft pitter-patter of rain drops dancing on the leaves, frozen in time with fox, deer, birds and raindrops alone in our own "church."

After a short while, a car passed us from behind, popping the bubble and restarting the hands of time. The fox jumped into the thick foliage and disappeared, the dear darted away and the chirping was replaced

Chapter 3

by tire noise. It was a peaceful moment I will never forget. When I was younger, my parents would read to me before bed. I loved *Goodnight Moon* and *This Is How Much I Love You*. The classics, but my dad would always find a way to work in this one story called *The Three Questions*. It told of an inquisitive boy who asked his animal friends the three most important questions of life: What is the most important time? Who is the most important person? What is the right thing to do?

I know it's a Tolstoy rip-off, but the message is the same and my church experience provided the answers. The most important time is always now. In the now, I can control what happens to the people, places and things in my immediate world. I can run harder, win the race, score the goal, solve the riddle and earn the A. The most important person is who's with me now, my soccer or track relay teammates or maybe just myself. The most important thing to do is always what's right: to help my teammates and friends, anyone in need and again, maybe just me.

The Zen-like experience I get from running is real. I admit that I sometimes hate running, especially when it's hot and muggy or when I didn't get enough sleep, yet I always feel proud and happy when I finish a run. The feeling is more than relief or even accomplishment, it's much more actually, it's therapeutic. One time my dad and I were arguing about something and it got pretty heated. He yelled at me, I yelled back and he yelled back even louder. I still had to go on my run, so being the sassy rebellious teenager that I am, I stomped up the stairs, got dressed and stormed out the front door. I ran the first five or six minutes angry, basically focusing on the argument and promising myself to stay mad at him. By the time I finished my run, my brain was focused on the pink cherry blossoms lining our street and how proud I was of my pace. I had completely forgotten about the argument and my promise to stay angry and when I walked back through the front door, the only emotion I felt was joy.

It's funny how the stress of running or playing any sport seems to counter and erase other stresses in life. The effect is immediate, like when your anger melts away, and is also long-lasting, like when you forget about the argument and instead tease your old man that his decrepit broken body could never keep up with you. I'm always nervous before a soccer game or race and sometimes before a practice. I get the exact same feeling before a test and in both situations, I use the same coping mechanism: numbers.

Numbers are comfortable. They're dependable and reliable. Whether prime, odd or even, the predictability of their relationships gives me control in situations where I feel out of control. There are infinite possibilities to explore with numbers, but in the end, there is always just one correct answer to any math problem. This movement from infinite to finite, from unknown to known is my source of comfort especially when playing with even numbers. Even numbers convey balance and equality, which is calming before a test or race. I remember being stuck in traffic while driving to an indoor meet in Virginia Beach. By the time we reached the track, my race had already started its first heat. I was in the last and as I ran into the stadium, I saw my heat lining up on the starting line and I began to panic. My head raced as I counted my steps and then the number of girls on the line. *8 total, 2, 4, 6, 8 = 1, 2, 3, 4 times 2, respectively. 4 times 2 is 8 and 8 times 100m is 800m, divided by 2 is 400m in 1 minute 10 seconds, 70 seconds total or 35 seconds each lap.*

My coach handed me my number as I ran past the check-in table and I stuck it to my hip. I threw my bag into the stands, ran onto the track, lined up with the other girls and took one big inhale before . . . *bang*! The gun fired and everyone exploded forward. In the few seconds it took me to run onto the track, I had calmed myself down just enough to focus on my race. Numbers became runners and then distance and finally time and with every step, literal and in my mind, the stress just disappeared. I use the same technique before a test, counting random things in the classroom until I get an even number. *3, 6, 9 window panes, shoot! Move to the other window. 12, 15, 18, good.* Now the stripes on my friend's glasses. *1, 2, 3, 4 times 2 sides is 8 total, I love the number 8. Even. Perfect.* My mind eases with the evenness of the room and I feel a sense of calm, like in my race. I know it's stupid and nonsensical and highly neurotic, but it's a system, it's my system and it works just as well in the classroom as it does on the starting line.

This may sound melodramatic, but I literally can't imagine my life without athletics. I can't imagine a life without running, without soccer, without competition, without sweat and without sports. I can't imagine dating someone who's not an athlete or at the very least athletic. I can't imagine not having a physical outlet, to sprint when I want to scream or crush the ball when I want to cry. Running and soccer have helped me so much physically and mentally. Whether I win or lose, whether I'm busted or bruised, I will never quit them as they have never quit me. They've made me strong and proud, they've given me an undying work ethic, a healthy Zen-like outlook and the confidence to overcome and achieve. In essence, a healthy body and mind.

Chapter 4

The Metamorphosis

Everything that changes need not be Kafkaesque.

Try telling that to an adolescent in the throes of puberty, with hair sprouting from the nether regions; acne erupting on their face, back and bum; body parts awkwardly bulging out in every direction and voices cracking like spring ice. Limbs become gangly, joints hurt for no reason and everything becomes a tripping hazard to the flippers that once were agile feet. Worst of all, the transformation occurs on center stage, framed by a spotlight amid a sea of heckling onlookers.

Franz Kafka's *The Metamorphosis* is often used metaphorically to describe puberty, a uniquely human trait first occurring in one of our earliest ancestors, *Homo erectus*, but not in non-human primates. The novella describes a man's horror to waking transformed into a giant insect, trapped in his bedroom and unable to communicate with his family. Consciousness and human awareness gradually drift away with his realization that the transformation is permanent. His death, however tragic, is a relief to his horrified family, who through inductive reasoning presume the bug's true identity. I personally prefer a caterpillar's analogy to the Kafkaesque spiral into revulsion and terror because what emerges from puberty is far from monstrous but pure strength and beauty, a mature adult of healthy body and mind.

Puberty evolved with changes in brain size and is a consequence of our watermelon-sized heads. The human brain-to-body ratio is the largest of all vertebrates except some whales, which also experience a prolonged adolescence and don't reach puberty until 6 to 13 years of age, depending on the species. Nothing in life or evolution is free, however, and we pay for this advantage by giving birth to the dumbest offspring with vertebrae. Human babies are born with disproportionately large but greatly undeveloped brains capable of little beyond sensing their environments and rudimentary motor control. Their brains are encased within a highly flexible skull composed of bony plates separated by membranous sutures and fontanelles, commonly called "soft spots," some of which close with bone growth after only a couple months while others take over two years to close. This provides the flexibility and protection to navigate the birth canal as well as room for the rapid brain growth that occurs in infants.

We continue to pay the evolutionary piper with prolonged parental care spanning multiple stages of childhood development including an adolescent phase that typically lasts five to eight years. All animals experience a period of sexual immaturity, but nothing as comparatively long as human infancy, childhood, juvenile and adolescent periods combined. Puberty starts later in boys and lasts slightly longer, although nutrition is the primary driver of timing regardless of sex. Genetics clearly play an important role, but body fat determines the threshold: too little and puberty is delayed, too much and it starts early. In fact, a byproduct of the obesity epidemic is early onset or precocious puberty. This can have serious long-term consequences like abnormal bone development and short stature due to premature closing of the growth plates in long bones. It can also cause several embarrassing developments like the formation of acne and facial hair in girls that, when combined with obesity-related body dysmorphia, can destroy a child's confidence and self-image.

Body fat regulates not only the timing of puberty but its rate and continues to control our ability to reproduce as adults. Female endurance athletes, for example, will often stop menstruating for months at a time, a phenomenon known as amenorrhea, once their body fat drops too low, usually below 18%. Low body fat due to excessive exercise can also delay the onset of puberty, which again can have serious long-term consequences that affect bone.

The Metamorphosis

Dr. Michael Levine, Chief emeritus of the Endocrinology and Diabetes division at the Children's Hospital of Philadelphia and my former mentor in Pediatric Endocrinology at Johns Hopkins, is an authority on calcium homeostasis and will fondly describe osteoporosis as a pediatric disorder. This disease results from bone demineralization or the loss of calcium and classically develops in postmenopausal women. However, bone mineral content is at its maximum when a woman is in her late 20s or early 30s and the rate of mineralization, when the addition of calcium is maximal, occurs during puberty. By the mid-30s, mineralization steadily declines and then plummets after menopause. These changes mirror those of estradiol (the principal estrogen produced by the ovaries) as the reproductive hormone prevents a particular type of bone cell, osteoclasts, from literally dissolving the bone matrix and releasing calcium into the blood. Thus, maximizing calcium and vitamin D intake as an adolescent and young adult is the best way to prevent osteopenia or osteoporosis that can develop later in life when estradiol levels are low to non-existent and osteoclast activity is high. In my house, girls always finish their milk!

The hormone leptin is the key regulator and connects nutritional intake with the reproductive system. It's produced by adipocytes, the cells that store fat, and its secretion increases as fat stores grow. Once in the bloodstream, it travels to the brain where, through a series of intermediates, it stimulates the release of the pituitary hormones that control reproduction: luteinizing hormone or "LH" and follicle stimulating hormone or "FSH." These hormones control both the ovaries and testes by stimulating production of the sex steroid hormones testosterone, estradiol and progesterone while also controlling development of mature eggs and sperm. Appropriately named LH also stimulates ovulation so when fat stores drop or don't develop, every aspect of reproduction is hampered or suppressed.

The reproductive system of girls and women is more susceptible to changes in body fat than it is in men simply because it demands more from energy reserves, although leptin controls reproduction equally in both sexes. In fact, I'm aware of a patient born with a mutated leptin gene who didn't produce the hormone. Leptin also stimulates satiety so as a young 20-something, he was obese with low muscle mass and no facial, axillary or pubic hair and had the penis and testes of a young boy. His endocrinologist started treating him with leptin injections and in one year, he became lean and mean, grew a beard, developed adult-sized genitalia, dropped his voice a couple octaves, got married and had hands-down the absolutely best year any man has ever had in the history of *Homo sapiens*!

Changes in reproductive hormone levels can have pretty dramatic effects on other physiological systems as well. The most well known of course are the anabolic effects of testosterone on muscle mass, which is really just the tip of the endocrine iceberg that develops during puberty. Why do adolescent girls develop curves? Because the adipocytes in hip, breast and butt depots respond to estradiol, increasing fat deposition, whereas adipocytes in other depots are insensitive to the hormone. Why do boys develop facial hair and larger muscles than girls? Because nearly all of the testosterone synthesized in ovaries—yes, girls and women make testosterone—is converted into estradiol through a chemical process known as "aromatization." Its gradual start, however, explains why girls in the early stages of puberty can develop facial hair or why hair on their arms and other places suddenly darken; increased steroid synthesis has begun, but aromatization has not.

Why are boys generally taller than girls? Could it be because testosterone stimulates bone growth or maybe that estradiol stimulates growth plate closure? Nope. A person's adult height is mostly dependent upon their height when puberty starts and not to differences in pubertal growth rates that are in fact identical in boys and girls and among different nationalities and demographic groups. This also explains the myth of tiny Asians and why second-generation children born from first-generation immigrants often tower over their parents. Within the confines of their genetic background, a young child's growth rate is dependent upon caloric intake. More food means more growth, resulting in a taller height when puberty begins. The earliest Asian immigrants to the United States moved from regions with comparatively low calorie intake like southern China, but once their children adopted an American high-calorie diet, the stereotypical differences in height between Asians and other nationalities disappeared. I once had a Gulliverian experience by boarding a plane in Hong Kong where at 5 feet 10 inches I'm taller than the vast majority of men and deboarding in Beijing to the surprise that I was now looking women eye to eye. Diets in the two regions are vastly different with Hong Kong consuming fewer calories on average and higher amounts of low-fat seafood whereas the Beijing diet is more "meat-n-potatoes."

These examples illustrate the extensiveness of pubertal changes to the adolescent body, how the intertwining of reproduction, nutrition and growth physiology are controlled by the endocrine system and how malnutrition, both under and over, can produce long-term health complications. Considering the complexity and degree of changes, it's no wonder why the metamorphosing body aches so much. Surprisingly, the injury rate of youth athletes before, during and after puberty is similar to that of young adults, although some adolescent tissues are particularly prone to injury simply due to the absolute or transitional differences in structure. Long bone growth plates, for example, are composed of soft cartilage in children and calcified bone in adults. The increased load of a rapidly growing and heavier body can sometimes turn what would have been a minor ankle sprain in a light young child or an adult with fully calcified bones into a broken leg in an adolescent. In fact, such injuries are far more common in adolescents than any other age group.

Larger bones and muscles also place larger loads on soft connective tissues, the elastic tendons connecting muscle to bones, the mostly inelastic ligaments stabilizing joints and the fibrous fascia that encases bone, muscle, skin and organs, holding them all in place. Osgood-Schlatter syndrome, another example, is extremely common among adolescent athletes and results from an inflamed insertion site of the patellar ligament, which connects the knee cap (aka patella) to the shin bone (aka tibia). This injury was falsely believed to occur more often in boys than girls but with the growth of competitive girls' sports, it is now known to occur equally among the sexes. Also well known is that the syndrome is self-limiting, meaning that it resolves on its own especially when the tibia growth plate closes. Why then do some orthopedists recommend invasive and expensive treatments like autologous-conditioned plasma or serum (ACP/S) therapy or platelet-rich plasma (PRP) injections when physical therapy with simple stretches and eccentric exercise will suffice? Do these treatments, ACP/S and PRP, really work? If so, why aren't they covered by health insurance? How else do the massive tissue remodeling and body sculpting that occurs with puberty affect the adolescent athlete and what should parents and athletes know about these metamorphosing bodies?

Coaches are always a rich source of information and as the principal person responsible for managing athletic injuries and overseeing the adolescent athlete's conditioning, it's important to know that they're almost always wrong. Most coaches understand the basics of RICE therapy—rest, ice, compression and elevation—for sprains and swelling, but that's about it. Most completely misunderstand even the basics of conditioning and exercise physiology and although at least some aspects like dynamic warm-ups are now common, most advice is based on outdated or inaccurate pseudo-science, inertia and misinformation. I've also never met a coach with a good understanding of the medical and health issues that are most pertinent to the adolescent athlete. Entire medical textbooks have been written on the topic and it's not my intention to rewrite said books. It's also not my intention to practice medicine because I'm wholly unqualified to do so. I am qualified, extremely well qualified in fact, to explain the underlying biology of important health care issues that impact adolescent athletes so that parents, athletes and coaches alike can make informed decisions that should always, always, *always* involve their pediatrician and often other medical specialists.

Pain Management "Dos and Don'ts"

Aches and pains, bumps and bruises, cuts and lacerations, sprains, breaks, tears, ruptures, contusions and concussions, injuries big and small, major and minor are all synonymous with sports. If you're going to play, at some point you're going to hurt.

The most commonly used therapeutics for treating pain and swelling due to inflammation, whether acute or chronic, belong to a class known as NSAIDs (pronounced "en-seds"), an acronym for nonsteroidal anti-inflammatory drugs. The word "nonsteroidal" is key as steroid hormones in the corticosteroid class like prednisone, which the liver activates by converting to prednisolone, are extremely potent anti-inflammatory drugs, but they don't squelch pain. They also can't be purchased without a prescription because they can do nasty things to a body when not taken correctly, producing maladies like muscle wasting, hyperglycemia and insulin resistance, growth retardation, cataract formation, obesity, osteoporosis, immunodeficiency and cognitive impairment just to name a few. These aren't *possible* reactions to the drug but *highly probable*. Corticosteroids evolved as the "off switch" for everything as generally retarding tissue growth and development preserves nutrients for the brain. The system coordinates the "fight and flight" response with acute stress, although chronic activation is nothing but damaging. Children are more sensitive to such nastiness and under no circumstances should they take prescription corticosteroids without supervision of a physician. Topical corticosteroids are great for treating mosquito bites and when corticosteroids are taken orally or inhaled, they help fight immune cell cancers and a plethora of autoimmune diseases. They can even extend the life of patients with Duchenne muscular dystrophy, but they're far too dangerous to be used without supervision. Going off the drug too soon, for example, can cause adrenal insufficiency where the adrenal glands completely stop functioning, causing anorexia and fatigue, nausea and vomiting, muscle and joint pain as well as severe drops in blood pressure that cause patients to faint and blood vessels to collapse.

Over-the-counter NSAIDs, by contrast, are excellent analgesics (pain relievers) that also fight inflammation. They're found in every medicine cabinet of every household and include aspirin, ibuprofen and naproxen sodium. Ibuprofen is more commonly known by its brand names Motrin® and Advil® and naproxen as Aleve®. Tylenol® is another analgesic and is known as acetaminophen in the United States and Japan and as paracetamol in most other countries. It too is ubiquitous to households, although it belongs to a different class of drugs and has a slightly different mechanism of action, which is an academic way of saying it does the same thing but in a different way.

Ibuprofen is the strongest of the four but has a half-life of only two hours. This means that half of the dose you take is gone, broken down by the liver and excreted into your urine after two hours whereas naproxen's half-life is over eight times longer. This is why many healthcare workers advise taking ibuprofen for acute pain, naproxen for chronic pain and alternating ibuprofen and acetaminophen every three hours for severe pain, swelling and fever. Aspirin is the weakest and is almost never given to children of any age due to its causative link with Reye's syndrome, a potentially fatal reaction to aspirin metabolites that can cause seizures, convulsions, repeated vomiting and liver failure.

Endurance athletes jokingly refer to ibuprofen as "vitamin I" because it's a favorite and all too frequently taken drug to treat the all too frequent muscle pain, inflammation and soft tissue injuries that are inherent to such sports. The cuteness of the joke is belied by the fact that ibuprofen is a drug, a real drug with known toxicities and serious side effects that, let's be honest, nearly all of us ignore. The drug has an excellent safety record in both children and adults and side effects are extremely rare when taken at proper doses, but people don't always follow directions and although it's tempting to assume that adults are better than children, this just isn't the case. Toxicities rarely occur at doses of 100 mg/kg or 45.5 mg/lb, which is the equivalent of a 100-pound child taking 23 tablets. This sounds like a lot because it is, yet ibuprofen overdoses among children are common and are responsible for 9% of all overdoses in adolescents, regardless of drug. Moreover, almost one-third of all overdoses with some type of pain reliever involved ibuprofen alone or in combination with other analgesics.

There are many reasons why children might overdose on what is normally a very safe over-the-counter drug. After all, it's available and familiar so the risk of unsupervised use is high. Adult dosing can be much higher than it is for children and any child taking adult doses would rapidly approach the toxicity threshold. Adolescents should never take over 1,200 mg/day while adult dosing maxes out at 3,200 mg/day, which is eerily close to the toxic threshold for children. Keep in mind that even recommended doses can have unwanted side effects like indigestion, nausea and constipation, which are among the most common. I have a dear friend who once complained of severe constipation that lasted for months. She survived the discomfort by taking laxatives and enemas until I learned she was self-medicating minor aches and pains with 800 mg ibuprofen four or five times a day, multiple days of the week. She luckily avoided the more serious reactions like gastrointestinal bleeding, ulcers and failing livers and kidneys, which are rare but potentially deadly. This nevertheless illustrates two extremely important points: never self-medicate—if you aren't a physician, ask someone who is—and always follow dosing instructions.

When taken as intended, all of these drugs are safe. When misused, they're also all dangerous. Studies indicate that ibuprofen is neither more nor less safe than other analgesics, and although the American Heart Association recommends that patients with cardiovascular disease use naproxen, the association also recognizes the benefit over other NSAIDs is likely negligible. Avoiding drug use altogether is obviously ideal and there are tangible ways to manage muscle pain or "DOMS" that don't involve chemistry.

DOMS is an acronym for delayed onset muscle soreness. It's a competitive athlete's nemesis, although I personally refer to it as "runner's bane" because distance runners suffer from it and spend more time and effort managing it than any other athlete. DOMS occurs after high-intensity and high-frequency training, which typically occurs during preseason conditioning for most sports and for most of a distance runner's season. The primary culprit is eccentric contractions, those that occur when muscles are stretched as this can literally rupture the muscle cell membrane and release a slew of different proteins and fluids outside the cell—imagine a water balloon with a tiny pinprick squirting water. The body responds by activating an inflammatory response that increases blood vessel permeability. Fluids carrying immune cells invade the damaged tissue, causing edema or swelling. These cells literally engulf the debris and then release inflammatory cytokines or hormones that attract more immune cells and activate muscle stem cells and the muscle repair process. That swelling and soreness you feel after pumping iron, the pain that causes marathon runners to walk backward down stairs for days following a race and the utter fatigue that prevents baseball pitchers from lifting their arm anywhere north of their shoulder, it's all due to DOMS.

Because distance runners and other endurance athletes are especially susceptible to DOMS, specific routines and exercises have been incorporated into their training programs to manage and avoid it. These include essential warm-up and cool-down routines to prepare the muscle, tendons and ligaments before a workout and to recover postworkout. Most coaches have learned to begin practices with task-specific dynamic stretches that are unique to the sport and to conclude practices with light static stretches. Some older coaches or parents who played in bygone eras will sometimes reverse the order by starting with static stretches or simply with a light jog, neither of which are sufficient. Studies have very convincingly shown that static stretching is too isolated to precondition the multiple tissues—muscle, tendon and ligaments—in multiple places and can even cause injury, either during the stretch or because the tissues weren't properly conditioned before exercise. Direct comparisons of the two programs further indicate that dynamic stretches can improve performance whereas static stretching can sometimes hurt it.

Static stretching consists of isolating a muscle or limb and slowly stretching it. Pretty simple, but pretty useless except for improving range of motion and flexibility. Dynamic stretching involves low-intensity movements like leg or arm swings and modified skipping. Track athletes are masters at dynamic stretches and will always start workouts, regardless of the planned intensity, with the same dynamic routines. Toe and heel walks; Frankensteins; butt kicks; high knees; A-, B- and C-skips; alternators and leg swings are common to every runner's warm-up routine, not only because they simultaneously condition all of the soft tissues needed for running but because they also reinforce proper running form and biomechanics. This is a very important and often overlooked benefit of dynamic stretching: it improves the biomechanics unique to the sport and in turn improves performance and . . . drumroll please . . . prevents injuries.

Warm-up routines for any sport involving running should start with a light jog followed by a dynamic stretching program that ends with sport-specific movements. If your coach isn't doing this, drop a hint or two or perform your own routine before the team activities start. YouTube is full of detailed examples and any reputable club or school program should have access to athletic trainers who can structure a sport-specific program on your or the team's behalf. Even sports like baseball can benefit greatly from dynamic routines that include jogging to increase circulation to the extremities followed by structured and sequential throwing drills that exercise the forearms (finger flexors) and wrist joint, rotator cuff and elbow, oblique and back muscles and then legs. Again, these routines not only properly condition the body for exercise but also reinforce proper form and prevent injuries.

Aches, pains and injuries will nevertheless develop even with proper warm-up and cool-down routines and NSAIDs, when properly taken, are reliable and safe, but taking them too much and too often increases risks for the myriad disorders mentioned earlier. Non-chemical treatments like cold exposure/cryotherapy and directed massage are in fact excellent alternatives to drugs and in some instances provide superior pain relief and counteract inflammation. Indeed, a recent meta-analysis of postexercise recovery techniques concluded that different types of massage and cryotherapy are most effective at treating DOMS.

Dr. Olivier Dupuy and other researchers in the Department of Sports Science, University of Poitiers, France, reviewed 99[1] studies that assessed different postexercise routines involving "active recovery"—low-intensity exercises that slightly elevate heart rate without stressing muscles—as well as massage, compression garments, different cryotherapies, static stretching and electrostimulation—stimulating muscle with light currents that activate tiny muscle twitches. Examples of active recoveries include easy jogs or "shakeout" runs, hurdle mobility stretches and low-intensity cycling (a personal favorite). Massage included foam rolling (another personal favorite) and other types of myofascial release, massage techniques that target inflamed, swollen and "knotted" areas in and around sore muscles. Wearing of compression garments was also studied as were cryotherapies like cold water immersion and use of cold chambers or cryocabins.

The least useful strategies were static stretching and muscle electrostimulation, which had no effect on DOMS or on addressing fatigue. Some studies even suggested that stretching can produce or exacerbate DOMS and although electrostimulation had a beneficial effect in a few studies, most reported no effect at all so the overall conclusion was ... *meh*.

By contrast, compression garments like socks, stockings and sleeves were found to improve both DOMS and fatigue. These garments are very similar to the stockings your grandparents use to treat poor circulation and prevent deep-vein thrombosis, which is the formation of blood clots usually in the lower legs. The garments work by compressing blood flow at a limb's farthest extreme, near the ankles and wrists, and gradually releasing pressure as blood rockets back toward the heart. The effect is like pinching the end of a garden hose: blood vessels swell on the upstream end of the compression, helping to clear out the muck from damaged muscle, and rocket toward the heart on the downstream end. It's crystal clear that they won't improve athletic performance yet they're pretty good at preventing and even treating DOMS.

The athletic garments are stylish, mine are a bright Miami turquoise, and have been rumored to improve athletic performance for years. In fact, manufacturers still make this claim despite a vast majority of clinical and academic studies indicating otherwise, studies performed by professors and university research scientists with MD and PhD degrees who quite appropriately are not paid by a sporting goods manufacturer. A few studies do indeed report minor improvements in performance. A few more demonstrate improvements in one or two abstract physiological processes, but not in athletic performance. Many if not most of these studies are underpowered, meaning they were performed using a small number of subjects while attempting to measure a large number of variables. This creates a data analysis nightmare where legitimate differences between study groups are hidden or apparent differences can't be trusted. It's the statistical equivalent of asking every girl in the school for a date. Eventually, someone says yes, but that doesn't mean she likes you and it certainly doesn't make you a player. In some instances, "P-hacking" may also have occurred. This is when data are analyzed to death and researchers accept the probabilities (hence "P") that fit their preconceived conclusions. You can probably guess what they do with those that don't.

Active recovery and cryotherapy similarly improved DOMS while cryotherapy also helped fight fatigue. Such benefits, however, came with caveats. Active recovery needed to be performed shortly after training or competing to be beneficial; anything beyond 24 hours had little impact and the recovery exercise needed to last long enough to get the heart pumping but couldn't be too long or too intense that it either exacerbated the extracellular buildup of metabolic waste or had no effect whatsoever. The benefit of cryotherapy depended to some degree on the specific type of therapy, whether cold exposure was alternated with warm exposure, the temperature involved and the time between exercising and treatment. As with active recovery, cryotherapy was only effective when performed shortly after exercising, within six hours, and muscles needed to be exposed to temperatures below 15°C/59°F. Exposure time was also critical with longer exposures have greater effects, although effective times were relatively short, lasting just 5 to 10 minutes and sometimes less.

The unequivocal champion of treatments, however, was massage therapy. In its many forms, massage increases blood flow, reduces edema and counters the inflammatory process at the molecular level. One of the molecules in question is muscle creatine kinase, an enzyme that leaches from injured muscle. Others include the stress hormone cortisol and several immune factors (e.g., IL-6, C-reactive protein, etc.) that directly activate tissue inflammation. It may sound fantastical, but all of these factors are reduced by massage therapy. In fact, the therapeutic efficacy of massage was first scientifically documented decades ago and has been practiced since before modern times. It may also explain the reflexive rubbing of injuries: why people from all corners of the earth, regardless of race, culture, class or indigenous status, will immediately grab and unconsciously rub an injured tissue.

Physically moving fluids away from the injured or affected area helps clear the molecular signals and alleviates the localized pressure. This in turn reduces swelling and pain. The analgesic effect may also be mediated by the production of beta-endorphins, the body's natural pain relievers that are produced with high-intensity exercise and with some massage therapies. Massage has even proven effective in alleviating DOMS and in particular pain among elite athletes competing in the Tor des Geants ultramarathon. Winners of this punishing race in the Italian and French Alps finish in 80 to 90 hours, cover a distance of 330 kilometers (205 miles) and climb a combined 24,000 meters (78,740 feet)!

Treatments need not last long, relatively speaking, as massages lasting 20 minutes provide significant relief from DOMS for over 24 hours. Some studies have even demonstrated a partial analgesic effect lasting up to 96 hours. The effect is transient, however, at least until the injured tissue is significantly repaired, which is why a routine to both prevent and treat soft tissue injuries incorporates many of these approaches. One of the most common techniques is foam rolling and is performed just as easily at home as it is on the field or in the gym. It can also be used in a warm-up routine, any time before dynamic stretches as well as after cool-downs. Limited studies further suggest that rolling is superior to neurodynamic therapy, a common approach used by physical therapists that isolates muscle movements controlled by a specific nerve.

There are many types of foam rollers. Some are smooth, some rough. Some have flat surfaces and others have grids like a tire. Some are soft, relatively speaking, and others look and feel like torture devices, although at least one study suggests that such differences are only cosmetic. The most common foam rollers are blue with a hard central core and a soft, flexible and textured surface. These are light and inexpensive but soften over time and most amateur marathoners will replace them a couple times a year. They're not composed of magical pixy dust so don't expect them to function like opioids. Instead, consider them as one of many tools to be incorporated into a standardized training schedule that when performed as follows will dramatically reduce the use of NSAIDs and prescription analgesics. Just remember that these tools can't replace the care of a good physician and physical therapist who will likely modify the recommendations listed here to fit your and your child's specific needs.

Recommendations to prevent and manage pain:

1. Start every warm-up routine with a very light jog lasting four to five minutes, possibly longer if the temperature is cold. Consider this "conversation pace" because you should be able to debate the complexities of life, dating in a modern interconnected world or the troubles with teenagers at will. The goal is to elevate your heart rate slightly and increase blood flow to the muscles. Stop when you've just started to sweat and if it's cold, stay bundled up for the next step.

2. Perform a generalized and then sport-specific dynamic stretching routine. Although it'll be tempting if working in a group, don't talk. Instead, focus on the biomechanics of the routine. Make your movements crisp and precise, exactly as instructed by your coach or trainer. This reinforces proper form and prevents injuries.
3. Use cryotherapy within the first one or two hours of an especially challenging workout or competition. Sitting in a bathtub with three to four inches of cold tap water and a bag of ice for five minutes works wonders for leg pain and prevents edema. Standing in a five-gallon bucket filled with ice-cold water is also good and less traumatic on the *unmentionables*. Shoulder and arm pain is similarly treated by attaching ice bags or cold packs to the area with ace bandages.
4. Wear appropriate compression garments immediately after the workout. They can also be worn before, after or in lieu of cryotherapy and although they look embarrassing, they're easily masked by whatever fashion suits you.
5. Form an intimate relationship with your foam roller. There are many effective techniques for rolling legs, butt and hip flexors and each can be done shortly before and within minutes of a workout. Because rolling prevents edema from returning, consider rolling a second time about 12 hours after a workout as well as on rest days. Back pain can be similarly managed by rolling with two tennis balls taped together. Examples of these exercises can be found on YouTube and many should be performed if cryotherapy can't.

If It Walks Like a Duck and Talks Like a Duck, It's a Chiropractor

I'll keep it short. Don't, just don't.

If you're interested in a more comprehensive discussion of chiropractors and the pseudo-science these non-doctors practice, I advise you to visit the chiropractor Wikipedia page. You'll find my contempt for the field and their practitioners to be commonly shared. You'll also find several references, which I encourage every snake oil believer to read, that discuss the metaphysical rather than scientific origin of "vertebral subluxation" and the uselessness of the chiropractic approach. I'll add that properly controlled clinical studies and comprehensive assessments of chiropractic studies by neutral arbitrators have never demonstrated most chiropractic practices to be effective. At best, some "adjustments" provide temporary relief of back and neck pain, likely through myofascial release, although the cost efficiency of treatments is questionable and many practices can be unsafe if performed without proper diagnosis and care of the injured tissue. This is contrasted by physical therapy, which is founded on sound anatomical and physiological science. Physical therapists also work in concert with orthopedists and sports medicine specialists and have training in biomechanics, trauma care and injury prevention. If you're interested in non-medicinal treatments for a sports-related injury, I implore you to avoid the chiropractic voodoo arts and instead visit a physical therapist.

Much of the confusion comes from a highly unlikely source, the National Institutes of Health who formed the Office of Alternative Medicine (OAM) in 1992 that was later changed to the National Center for Complementary and Alternative Medicine and more recently to the National Center for Complementary and Integrative Health. The fluidity in titles was paralleled by leadership changes as real scientists ran the entity as one would expect: scientifically. This didn't sit well with the politicians who founded the OAM, Senator Tom Harkin and Representative Berkley Bedell, both from Iowa. Harkin believed bee pollen supplements cured his hay fever while Bedell believed cow colostrum—the antibody-laden first milk every mammal produces shortly after giving birth—cured his Lyme disease. No, I'm not making this up and no, neither political party, Democratic nor Republican, has a monopoly on the conspiracy market of nonsense.

Bedell and particularly Harkin grew increasingly frustrated over the Office/Center's failures to *prove* the effectiveness of alternative approaches and Harkin expressed this frustration in a 2009 Senate hearing on integrative healthcare, saying, "One of the purposes of this center was to investigate and validate alternative approaches. Quite frankly, I must say publicly that it has fallen short. I think quite frankly that in this center and in the office previously before it, most of its focus has been on disproving things rather than seeking out and approving."

I doubt Harkin understood how exquisitely he shot his own foot with this comment while simultaneously demonstrating an utterly incompetent understanding of how science is practiced. Not only did he publicly, unexpectedly and unknowingly yet very accurately criticize the entire field of alternative medicine, highlighting its failures and validating the scientific community's critique of its woolly minded underpinnings, he also expressed a common misunderstanding of the scientific method: that experiments are performed to *prove* something. This is how propaganda is practiced, not science, which serves only to *determine* and never to prove. The data are what they are whether or not you like or dislike the outcome and, in this case, Senator Harkin was clearly in the dislike camp.

Before and since Harkin's comment, countless studies tested and challenged the central tenets of alternative medicine in attempts to determine the efficacy and safety of various practices and as Harkin admits, the results were and are disheartening to the snake oil believers. This includes vertebral subluxation and other manipulations and treatments performed by chiropractors and similar purveyors of alternative medicine, like acupuncture and its Western derivative dry needling. Many of these studies report positive effects on pain relief, stroke recovery, constipation, depression, nasopharyngeal carcinoma, premenstrual syndrome or anything else a hypochondriac could fear. In fact, it's difficult to find a malady, discomfort, disorder or disease that isn't treatable by acupuncture and this should raise red flags from even the least skeptical of us. Miracle cure-alls don't exist.

The problem isn't the lack of clinical results but the lack of believable and reproducible results due to how the studies were performed, usually without proper controls. Studies often weren't blinded, meaning that study subjects, the scientists running the studies or both were fully aware of what was being done, to whom it was being done and how much was being done. When studies were controlled for such placebo effects, most significant differences are lost. This is especially true when sham groups are included. A "sham" control is one that replicates the treatment in a way that shouldn't elicit a response. With acupuncture, this could involve placing the needles in the wrong place or not deep enough or with electroacupuncture, attaching the electrodes but not activating the current. If a sham control and treatment have similar effects, the treatment is ineffective and any response is due to surveyor bias, subject expectations or weird luck, but not to the treatment.

Believers of acupuncture will argue vociferously that sham controls are meaningless because they themselves have effects, but this illustrates precisely the point of using experimental controls. Jabbing needles into a living tissue has an effect, multiple effects actually, and these all must be controlled. Otherwise, there's no way to determine if the treatment—the accurate insertion of needles to influence the mythical power of qi—has an appreciable effect on a subject's physiology or, alternatively, that the generalized insertion of said needles in non-specific places weakly alters local inflammatory responses, the release of endorphins or even peripheral nerves located in the affected area. Who knows? Nobody, that's who, because the hypothetical mechanisms by which acupuncture or any other chiropractic treatment supposedly work is enigmatic to scientists and to chiropractors alike.

TREATING "SHIN SPLINTS" AND OTHER TENDINOPATHIES

Shin splints, that annoying pain running along the inside of one if not both shins, the piercing feeling of an ice pick into your leg as you first step out of bed in the morning, the pain that literally hurts with every single step forcing you to gingerly walk as flat-footed as possible, this is shin splints.

The medical term for shin splints is "medial tibial stress syndrome" and it is one of the most common injuries among runners and jumpers. The injuries are classified as tendinopathies because despite the name, the shin or tibia isn't injured. Rather, shin splints result from injuries to the musculoskeletal system of the tibialis anterior or "TA" muscle, specifically to the tendons that connect the TA to the top of the tibia bone and to the medial cuneiform bone of the foot. The TA lifts the toes up, keeping the foot in a dorsiflexed position, but also flexes to absorb the force of a foot plant on landing. Shin splints result from overuse and are especially common among new runners and jumpers and among weekend warriors reliving their glory days. The damaged tissue becomes inflamed and swelling spreads along the space separating the soft tissue from bones, which complicates locating the actual injury site as pain often diffuses along with the swelling and can cover a wide area. It also complicates treatment because these spaces are not well vascularized and analgesics like ibuprofen don't easily reach them, which explains why the drugs are only weakly effective.

Tendinopathies are by far the most common class of running or running-related injuries. Approximately 80% of running injuries are tendinopathies and recent studies of distance runners suggest that 40 to 45% will annually suffer from a tendinopathy somewhere in the leg, which is known as the injury prevalence, whereas the incidence of new injuries is remarkably similar. The fact that the prevalence and incidence are the same means that the occurrence of these injuries is static. This should inspire a collective "hmmm" because it means that all the technological advances in shoe design and the myriad medical devices developed to treat shin splints, like compression sleeves, calf braces, crosstraps, orthotic insoles and arch supports, have had little effect. As I discuss shortly, some have even been tested in controlled clinical trials and based on these results, they have the identical efficacy as sacrificing small animals while chanting prayer mantras to Phil Knight, the loveable and eccentric co-founder of Nike.

Shin splints are the second most common tendinopathy of all ages and the most common among adolescent athletes. The latter are believed to be more susceptible to developing shin splints because the growth of elastic tissues in muscle, the tendons and connective tissues, lags behind that of muscle fibers. Imagine a game of tug-of-war between two NFL linemen. As long as the rope is strong enough, someone eventually pulls the other over a line and "work" is performed. This is analogous to muscle pulling on bone to affect movement. Now imagine those linemen pulling on kite string.

The rapid growth of muscle and bone during puberty is eventually compensated with elastic fiber growth and as long as proper form and warm-ups are performed, shin splints disappear for most adult athletes that don't suffer from the "overs": overtrain, overexert, overuse and overdo it. The injury is avoidable but not predictable, although careful examination of running form, limiting downhill running, use of easy shakeout runs and rest days along with proper running shoes with good fore- and mid-foot support are essential. Remember that the TA absorbs force when the front of the foot hits the ground so rapid decelerations and long downhill running require the TA to produce greater forces than gradual decelerations and running on flat surfaces. Proper running shoes absorb and distribute energy, requiring less work by the TA, and proper running form without dramatic heal striking and "foot slap" also lessen the TA's workload and potential for injury. In fact, shin splints can be avoided by following these guidelines.

1. Start and conclude practices with barefoot jogging to strengthen the TA and build flexibility into the lower leg.
2. Follow barefoot jogging with a structured warm-up routine composed of sport-specific dynamic stretches.
3. Limit the TA's workload by spreading out exercises with high workload demands, such as hill running and plyometrics.
4. Never decelerate rapidly when training, embrace the "run through" philosophy.
5. On "off" days or after recovering from practice, perform calf raises (up and down on your toes), preferably on the edge of a stair, to increase calf muscle and Achilles tendon flexibility.
6. Wear proper shoes. Conditioning should be performed in high-quality running shoes and practicing in a sport-specific shoe so buy multiple shoes and use them conditionally. Gradually converting to "low-drop" running shoes may help athletes with significant heal strike to avoid shin splints by gradually training the TA. Key words here are "gradual" and "may" because rapidly converting to a low-drop shoe can actually cause shin splints if the workload demand (e.g., hill running) is high.

Taping and other forms of compression can work for some tendinopathies, just not for shin splints. They provide minimal and temporary relief at best and are short lived with exercise. Indeed, modern athletic trainers and physical therapists don't advocate use of compression devices for shin splints, yet some coaches and several websites will tell you different. The former are usually from bygone eras when such practices had yet to be disproven while the latter are simply taking advantage of injured athletes desperate for relief. Both should be ignored.

Some tendinopathies can be treated with isometric eccentric exercises. Isometric means "equal dimensions" so isometric exercises are those where muscles contract but don't shorten. Hanging from a chin-up bar, pushing against a wall or holding a dumbbell in place are good examples. Eccentric exercises are those that occur with stretched muscle and should be performed with care. Muscle is at its most fragile state when stretched so these exercises are performed with small loads, either with very low weights or with none at all. The idea is to strengthen the muscle without stressing the elastic fibers, hence no shortening, and clinical studies indicate these exercises appear to work well for some but not all tendinopathies. Unfortunately, this approach has not been shown to work with shin splints and although "rest, stretch and ease back into it" is the typical treatment approach of most physicians, exercise physiologists and physical therapists have devised the following superior approaches that work quite well when combined.

1. Ice the lower leg by standing in ice water or strapping ice/cold packs to the affected area. Never apply heat. Allowing the leg/area to warm to room temperature before again applying the cold therapy will help increase circulation through the area and may eventually hasten recovery.
2. Take your favorite NSAID to lessen the pain and to suppress the chemical signals that cause inflammation.
3. Frequently massage the medial edge of the TA, the side adjacent to the tibia bone. Start above the inflamed area and extend past it. Fingers and thumbs work well, but hand-held rolling sticks work best. This is a form of myofascial release and helps clear fluid from the inflamed area.
4. Use a foam roller and calf raises (if not too painful) to increase flexibility of the plantar flexors, the muscle system that pulls the toes down and acts counter to the TA.

Chapter 4

About a dozen clinical trials with athletes or soldiers have studied other somewhat controversial treatment strategies for shin splints. These include using sound waves, either ultrasound or extracorporeal shockwaves; transdermal (through the skin) drug delivery aided by electrical current or ultrasound otherwise known as iontophoresis and phonophoresis/sonophoresis, respectively; and periosteal pecking or dry needling of bone (ugh!). Some studies report a minor but positive effect on pain, although critical reviews of these studies not surprisingly characterized them as "low quality." Other therapies incorporating low-energy lasers (seriously?!?) and physical supports like leg braces or compression socks were also studied and were found to have no benefit whatsoever. These strategies are in my opinion the technology equivalents of a Hail Mary pass. They lack any semblance to underlying physiological justification and although they're relatively inexpensive, animal sacrifices and mantra chanting would again work just as well. One of the more common treatments for tendinopathies, however, is very expensive, is not covered by health insurance and is peddled by even respectable orthopedists yet it again lacks sound physiological justification and has even been proven ineffective in large clinical trials: platelet-rich plasma injections or "PRP."

This therapy became famous when Tiger Woods used it to treat tears to his lateral collateral ligament and Achilles tendon. Its success met great media fanfare and is touted in almost every orthopedic clinic in the country as Tiger's name is dropped daily in pursuit of profits. Rarely mentioned, however, is the fact that Tiger was also treated with corrective surgery or that a multitude of clinical studies have failed to demonstrate the therapy to be effective. To date, 60 meta-analyses of studies featuring PRP for treating a variety of injuries have been published in addition to about 1,500 individual studies of PRP treatments of the knee and ankle injuries, yet the scientific and medical community remains skeptical. Publications by orthopedists who regularly advocate for and perform the treatments not surprisingly report an effect, although many meta-analyses describe these studies as low-quality with high risk for bias, which is science speak for saying, "It might not be crap, but it ain't good."

Most studies find the treatment to be safe but utterly ineffective and when reviews are limited to high-profile assessments published in the finest medical journals with the strictest oversight and most rigorous standards, the waters start to clear. The *Journal of the American Medical Association*, commonly known as *JAMA*, for example, has published three clinical trial studies of PRP treatment for musculoskeletal diseases including knee and ankle osteoarthritis as well as Achilles tendinopathy. I'd like to summarize the authors' conclusions, but I think it's best to let them speak for themselves.

> *Intra-articular injection of PRP, compared with injection of saline placebo, did not result in a significant difference in symptoms or joint structure at 12 months. These findings do not support use of PRP for the management of knee [osteoarthritis].*[2]

> *Intra-articular PRP injections, compared with placebo injections, did not significantly improve ankle symptoms and function over 26 weeks. The results of this study do not support the use of PRP injections for ankle osteoarthritis.*[3]

> *"Among patients with chronic Achilles tendinopathy who were treated with eccentric exercises, a PRP injection compared with a saline injection did not result in greater improvement in pain and activity."*[4]

There's no convincing evidence that PRP works for treating tendinopathies or most other injuries or diseases. However, it's clear that the treatment is safe and this is why the FDA allows orthopedists to perform it. Note that I didn't say the treatment is "approved" by the FDA because it isn't. Instead, the FDA has approved laboratory procedures for isolating platelets to be used in bone graft procedures and because PRP has nothing to do with bone grafts, the therapy is considered "off label" and insurers won't pay for it. This means that if you're interested in trying Tiger's expensive and unproven therapy with a long and well-documented history of failing in the clinic, one that hasn't received FDA approval and is based on flawed basic science, you better have deep pockets. Alternatively, you could set up the mouse traps, light some candles and start summoning Phil Knight.

PREVENTING PAIN FROM PREVENTING ACNE
Pimples don't make you run slower. They don't make your muscles and joints hurt and they can't cause you to lose games or races. The most commonly prescribed medication for acne, however, will.

Isotretinoin is sold under many different trade names including Amnesteem®, Claravis®, Myorisan®, Sotret®, Zanatane® and especially Accutane®. It has a structure very similar to vitamin A and was developed over 60 years ago to treat different types of skin cancer. In fact, it's still used in treating squamous cell carcinoma and certain types of skin lymphomas, but not melanoma. It's also used to treat different skin inflammatory conditions like psoriasis and rosacea and can address excessive oiliness, although it is primarily approved for severe or resistant acne. It works by inhibiting the skin's sebaceous glands, decreasing their size and the amount of oil that they secrete. Less oil means fewer clogged pores and a clear complexion.

The drug works extremely well, too well actually, and produces a long list of side effects. This is indeed a serious drug that can produce potentially very serious adverse reactions. Although they occur rarely to very rarely, the drug should always be used under supervision of a dermatologist and if taken by a young or adult woman, an obstetrician should also advise. Children are usually not treated with isotretinoin until after puberty because it prematurely closes the growth plates in bone, which causes short stature, and bone demineralization, which increases the risk of osteopenia. Moreover, any reproductive-capable female, adolescent girls or adult women, is required to simultaneously use two forms of birth control when taking isotretinoin. This usually involves condoms in combination with oral contraception or intra-uterine devices because isotretinoin interferes with fetal neural development and can cause severe birth defects during pregnancy. In fact, girls and women who do become pregnant while taking isotretinoin are strongly advised to immediately abort the pregnancy.

Dry lips and skin are among the most common side effects. Athletes and runners are particularly likely to suffer from dry cracked lips because the heavy breathing from running already dries the lips. For this reason, most coaches advise runners to always carry lip balm, which is a necessity for athletes taking isotretinoin. Myalgia and arthralgia or muscle and joint pain, respectively, are also quite common side effects of taking isotretinoin and are caused by the same mechanisms responsible for the birth defects: vitamin B9 and folate deficiency.

In a developing embryo, folate is critical for a process known as neural tube closure, which gives rise to the brain and spinal cord. Anything that lowers folate levels in an embryo or even during fetal development can produce a variety of horrible abnormalities in the brain and spinal cord. Conversely, supplementing with folic acid, which is converted to folate in the body, can prevent these defects and is universally recommended by obstetricians.

Folate is used to produce the amino acid methionine, the most critical of all amino acids because almost every single protein in the human proteome, in fact in almost every cell of every living organism, starts with the amino acid methionine. Proteins are constructed like a string of pearls with individual amino acids serving as individual pearls that are added in sequential order. Without methionine, the string/protein is never made. Methionine is synthesized via a biochemical pathway that ultimately converts a molecule called homocysteine into methionine. This conversion requires folate so when folate levels are low, tissue levels of homocysteine rise and this precursor crystalizes in the elastic fibers of muscle and on the articular surfaces of bone joints. The resulting pain and discomfort is normally not severe, but it is significant enough to bench an athlete. NSAIDs, myofascial release and cryotherapy are useless against the pain, although there is a simple and highly effective treatment: oral supplementation with folic acid and vitamin B12.

It's surprising that this remedy is not standard of care for acne patients taking isotretinoin and I'm amazed that many dermatologists are unaware of its effectiveness especially as oncologists regularly advise taking the supplements when their patients are treated with isotretinoin. Before you jump on the "doctors are money-grubbing materialists disinterested in cheap over-the-counter solutions" bandwagon, you should know that there have only been 11 studies published to date that even address the issue and only one specifically studied muscle and joint pain. Nevertheless, evidence supporting the remedy's effectiveness is strong despite its relative paucity and dosing recommendations have even been established.

Both folic acid and vitamin B12 are available as oral supplements. They're inexpensive and can be found in most grocery, pharmacy and nutrition stores. The doses used in clinical trials of folic acid varied significantly from 0.5 mg/day to 5.0 mg/day and vitamin B12 was administered orally or by infrequent injections. Taking two folic acid pills of 800 mcg or 1,330 mcg DFE daily and one vitamin B12 pill of 3,000 mcg every other day would approximate the doses used to suppress muscle and joint pain. I've used this dosing with athletes I've trained and it was incredibly successful with no adverse reactions. This is consistent with the results obtained in clinical trials and in most cancer clinics. In the one study that specifically addressed muscle and joint pain, all subjects reported improvements after just one week of treatment and were completely pain free well before the study ended at six weeks.

So talk to your dermatologist, take your vitamins and get back on the field, pitch, track, road or wherever it is you play!

MEILANI'S TAKE (16 YEARS OLD)

Moral ambiguity aside, playing the Coyotes' way with extreme aggression produced an occasional injury as well as an *often* injury and an *always there* injury. It's ironic that despite our extreme aggression and mascot, the Coyotes were a team of mostly short, thin players who at any given time were injured. The other teams seemed bigger and stronger, but they were never as fast or aggressive (dirty?) as the Coyotes and I always wondered if they were as hurt by the end of the game as we were. We had broken arms, feet, fingers and toes. Stress fractures and sprained ankles, a personal favorite, were common, and concussions were a rite of passage. Most of my non-soccer or non-Coyote friends never had a serious injury. By the time I was 15, I experienced six sprained ankles, a broken foot and a broken wrist. I sprained one ankle on a long run (stupid chestnuts) and re-sprained the same ankle warming up for a track meet. Everything else happened in soccer.

My first serious injury started simple enough yet snowballed across sports and seasons. I was just messing around with friends playing a small game of possession, wearing the wrong shoes in an overgrown field, when I took a wrong step and twisted my ankle in a hidden hole. In just a few minutes, my ankle swelled to the size of a tennis ball, a few minutes later a softball. The swelling then began creeping up my leg and I started freaking out.

Everyone asked about the physical pain, but this was brief and after the second ankle sprain, I learned to ignore it. I instead thought of the setback, how my hard work was wasted and how much more work would be needed. Getting injured was kind of fun when I was younger. Friends thought I was tough, parents gave me special attention and teachers gave me special privileges. As I got older, the attention and privileges started to feel like pity and I experienced the true pain of injury: feelings of helplessness, despair and anguish. I've learned that playing at a competitive level is a double-edged sword. You start relying on it as much as the team relies on you and when it's gone, your whole life falls out of balance. When I was angry, I ran. When I was sad, I ran. When I was happy, I ran. Without the outlet of exercise, I began to feel useless and lazy, stuck in a cycle of self-pity.

I was a rising freshman when it happened and soccer tryouts were just two months away. I could *not* get injured I thought. For a week RICE—rest, ice, compression and elevation—ruled my days. I then started physical therapy. For two weeks, we worked on increasing circulation and regaining flexibility and for the next six weeks building strength in the lateral leg muscles and butt or "glutes." The physical therapist finally released me to practice with a warning: "take it easy and take it slow."

Practicing for the first time in over six weeks felt amazing! I was fast and strong again albeit a little wobbly. All those days of sitting around feeling sorry for myself were over. At the very end of practice, my coach decided to reward us with a game of world cup where you and your partner try to score against all the other teams crowded around the goal. I clearly wasn't playing my best yet my team made the finals and I had scored most of the goals. I was excited, I was anxious to start and I was focusing on my opponents when a girl watching from the sidelines shot the ball toward the goal, shanking it and accidentally hitting my foot. I didn't see it coming and, in a flash, I was on my back clutching my re-sprained ankle.

I was so angry. I was angry at her. I was angry at the ball. I was angry at my stupid ankle. Mostly I was angry at myself. *Why am I always trying to rush everything? Why didn't I just skip practice?*

I didn't say a word on the ride home. As soon as my dad pulled into the garage, I burst into tears not because of the pain but because the weeks of recovery were wasted time. Everything would need to be repeated. Worst of all, I would miss varsity tryouts.

A few days later, while I was wallowing in despair and self-pity, I received some incredible and unexpected news, a stroke of tragedy and luck that changed my life: soccer tryouts and the entire season were delayed due to COVID-19. I know it sounds horrible, but I was happy. I wasn't happy for the pandemic, I mean I'm not a horrible person, I was just happy to find a silver lining in the tragedy.

This time I didn't rush my body. I didn't rush anything but "took it easy and took it slow." I worked with my physical therapist three times a week and daily by myself. I thought about my mistakes, about luck in general and about how much I love soccer and running and what they mean to me. I would sometimes complain about waking up early to run or practicing in bad weather and didn't realize how much I actually loved both until they were gone. I missed all of the aches, pains, sweat and stress that come with running and soccer and looking back, I can't believe it took six sprained ankles to realize how sports have become the foundation of my happiness.

Chapter 5

Pink or Blue?

So how old were you when you chose to be straight? Had you chosen your gender or sexual identity yet or did you reserve this watershed moment for a grandiose reveal?

In *Homo sapiens*' 300,000-year existence, give or take 10,000 or 15,000 years, nobody has ever chosen their sexual orientation or gender identity. Neanderthals maybe, but not us. Modern patients with ambiguous genitalia or gender dysphoria might have chosen gender-affirming care that revised a few birth certificates and wardrobes, but the patients' gender identities were hardwired from well before birth. Anyone who believes that children choose to be society's pariah, to be tormented and bullied by the Neanderthals among us, to be outcasts from their families and tortured by their reflection is ignorant, intolerant or evil. Yes, I have an opinion on the issue and no, you probably don't know where I'm going with this, but you should be assured that my objectivity is founded on thousands of peer-reviewed publications written by the world's authorities on developmental, reproductive and behavioral biology. These were informed by decades of biomedical and zoological research and by modern medical science. My opinion, which will come soon enough, may be subjective, but not the underlying facts. These are non-debatable.

1. Gender identity and sexual orientation are related yet different and independent.

2. Homosexuality and bisexuality are natural, commonly occurring in most/all animal systems.
3. Sex results from a process, not a thing.

Gender identity is whether a person considers themselves to be male or female. It usually aligns with the presence or absence of the male Y chromosome, but not always, and although the outcome is assumed to be binary, some individuals can't tell because what they see in the mirror doesn't match how they feel inside while others recognize the ambiguity and embrace intergender or intersexuality, legitimate umbrella classifications for non-binary individuals. It's not black and white but a whole lot of gray.

Sexual orientation refers to the sex of attraction: heterosexuality, homosexuality and bisexuality. It can be difficult to define as, for example, in prisons where homosexual acts are committed by persons who strongly consider themselves to be heterosexual. This presents a conundrum for psychologists and neuroethologists studying the behavior as the subject's definition of sexual orientation is strongly influenced by culture and experiences. This is resolved using questionnaires to sample behaviors, fantasies and attractions that together define a subject's true sexual orientation objectively that quite often doesn't match the subject's own definition. The prisoner's situation is a prime example. Consider also a person who transitions from male to female yet was always physically attracted to women. Did this person's sexual orientation also change from heterosexual to homosexual or did society's perspective?

Although distinctly independent traits, gender identity and sexual orientation are obviously related, not only psychologically but also by the genetic, biochemical and physiological processes that control their development. The traits' underlying natural basis *shouldn't* surprise anyone yet I wouldn't be writing on the topic if it didn't. Disbelievers and believers alike are encouraged to read what is quite possibly the most riveting book on the topic *As Nature Made Him: The Boy Who Was Raised as a Girl* by John Colapinto. I won't play spoiler other than to say that no matter how hard fraudulent scientists tried or cooked their data, no matter what physical, chemical and emotional abuses the boy's parents and caregivers performed, nothing, absolutely nothing could change his gender identity or sexual orientation. It simply wasn't a matter of choice even after the accidental and intentional atrocities were committed.

Plasticity in sexual orientation is also very well documented in nature and in domestic animals. In fact, homosexuality—defined simply as sexual acts between individuals of the same sex—occurs in most households, kennels and dog parks. Honestly, who hasn't witnessed male dogs humping one another? One may question whether the motivation behind male dogs mounting one another or male dolphins orally stimulating one another or dominant male sea lions anally penetrating subordinate males, which also occurs among African lions and many other mammals, mirrors that of human homosexuals. One could, but one would be missing the point and risking anthropomorphizing the acts, each of which has an evolutionary explanation that may or may not be consistent with the human experience. They are nevertheless sexual acts performed on and between individuals of the same sex.

If you really want your mind blown, consider natural examples of transexual animals like marine polychaete worms that change sex several times in life, sharing the high maternal burden of reproduction, or the 500-plus species of sexually plastic fishes. This includes protandrous species that all start as male before changing to female, a process initiated by the appropriate environmental and social triggers. Protogynous species start as female and change to male also when triggered. In all of these species, a particular individual's sex is determined genetically while triggering induces a change in the expression of genes that mimic those involved in human sexual development. These genetic experiments have only been performed in a few species, but it's highly likely that nearly identical changes in gene expression occur in most if not all sexually plastic fishes. If your mind still isn't blown, note that the sex change process can be manipulated by the anti-depressant Prozac and that wastewater containing small quantities of anti-depressants are known to interfere with the reproductive cycles of wild fish.

My last and favorite example proving quite convincingly that sexual orientation and sexual identity are indeed natural phenomena comes from the farm. Dr. Fred Stormshak, Distinguished Professor of Animal

Science at Oregon State University, has documented homosexual behavior as well as the underlying anatomical and biochemical basis of male-oriented rams. On average, 8% of domestic rams demonstrate exclusive male-oriented preference with 60 to 70% demonstrating exclusive female orientation. The remaining never worry about spending a Saturday night alone or are asexual.

Homosexual behaviors in sheep were first identified in field studies of Rocky Mountain bighorn sheep. Ranchers and farmers, however, have likely been well aware of it for centuries and respectively refer to female- and male-oriented rams as "studs" and "duds." Mounting between males is often used to establish dominance, which doesn't reflect mate preference and is in ways analogous to some same-sex interactions in prisons, so true male-oriented preference was established by simply giving the duds a choice: 6 to 10% chose male.

Dr. Charles Roselli of the Oregon Health Science University and former trainee of Dr. Stormshak has continued the work and has described developmental mechanisms that change brain structures consistent with the behavior. Most importantly, these changes occur *before* rams become sexually active and can even be detected in fetal lambs. Coincidentally, these structures match those documented in brains of human male homosexuals and can be experimentally induced in rodents and other mammals with carefully timed hormone treatments. Timing is critical because the brain's hormone sensitivity window is only open at early stages of fetal development and once it's closed, the reproductive hormones testosterone and estradiol have no effect, at least not on the neural development that influences sexual orientation or gender identity.

It should be noted that several pivotal studies have documented brain structures of transgender people that match their "chosen" gender rather than their genotypic sex. This is true for male-to-female and female-to-male transsexuals and includes different neural regions well known to influence sexual orientation and gender identity, regions like the bed nucleus of the stria terminalis or "BSTc" and the interstitial nucleus of the anterior hypothalamus or "INAH." These easily forgettable terms are mentioned only to emphasize one very important point: details matter. Details demonstrating an anatomical basis for gender dysphoria, details demonstrating conservation between human and animal studies and details demonstrating support between genetic and *in vivo* neural imaging studies, all of which demonstrate a neurobiological origin for gender identity and gender dysphoria.

In other words, gender identity, whether in trans- or cisgender people, is never chosen but results from the growth, connectivity, molecular biology and biochemistry of neurons within specific brain regions. It also cannot be established with hormone therapy, social clues, environmental pressures or—I can't believe I'm writing this –children's books!

Assessing gender identity in animals is in many ways easier than in people. People are usually but not always candid in surveys even when their identity is protected, so although you can't simply ask a ram, bluehead wrasse, zebrafinch or hyena—all incredibly fascinating models of sexual development and plasticity—if they identify as male, female or intersex, you can watch for sexually dimorphic behavior patterns. These are easily quantifiable behaviors that are uniquely expressed by one sex or the other and although the duds displayed some aspects of female sexual behavior, specifically male orientation, other sexually dimorphic behaviors remained male. They hadn't transitioned to female but retained their male gender identity.

Female spotted hyenas are even more fascinating. They're much larger than males and display typical male pattern behaviors for mammals like aggression and dominance. They also rule their matriarchal clans and have ... wait for it ... an enormous masculinized pseudo-penis to match their masculinized brains and behaviors. Their sexual orientation remains heterosexual, but their gender identity, at least from typical mammalian perspectives, has transitioned to male. I know I'm nerdin' out again, but you have to admit this is all very, very cool!

All of this illustrates the power of nature to mold two of the three pillars of sex: gender identity and sexual orientation. The third pillar, gender roles, is defined by social networks and culture. Boys like blue, wear pants and play with trucks. Girls like pink, wear dresses and play with dolls. Such roles are nurture-dependent and although some may reinforce behaviors with strong genetic roots, they are easily overruled by social pressures. I wore Speedos as a kid, but when my family moved to a distant community, I was teased for wearing bikini bottoms on my first visit to the town's pool. My social network changed as did the social pressures that defined gender roles in my community and as a result, I started wearing cutoff blue jeans.

This brings us to the nature versus nurture debate. The first and only rule of the debate is that there is no debate. That's right, you've been hoodwinked by Hollywood, fake news and pseudo-scientists into believing nonsense. Science has never really debated the issue, especially in modern times as the heritability of behaviors was well understood even before Darwin's treatise. Instead, science has debated the relative degree of nature versus nurture, recognizing that all behaviors are influenced by both genetics and the environment. Think of every behavior as falling on a continuum with "closed genetic programs," which is science speak for nature, on one end of the continuum and "open genetic programs" or nurture on the other. Some behaviors are strongly influenced by genes and fall closer to the closed side while others are strongly influenced by environment and fall closer to the open side.

Baby spiders, for example, will grow up to construct webs identical to their mother's as long as they eat properly. Web-building behavior in these species is a relatively closed genetic program, but not entirely as it's also influenced by food availability. Lovebirds carry nest building materials in their beaks or tucked under their tailfeathers. Crossing beak-with tail-carriers produces a neurotic bird that can't make up its mind, constantly tucking and untucking material from its tail. I once debated the genetic basis of behavior with a famous albeit somewhat close-minded scientist who helped map the dog genome. He dogmatically (pun intended) insisted that all behaviors were genetic in origin and that environment had no influence whatsoever. We were watching his border collie chase a tennis ball, responding to his commands to move left and right, stop and go. I responded by asking what would happen if every time he commanded the dog to move right, I smacked its head with a baseball bat: a crude but effective mic-drop. Now consider LGBTQ people living in ostracizing communities, unforgiving or even violent to their mislabeled "lifestyle choices," and you can understand why they might suppress their closed genetic programs governing sexual orientation or move to more enlightened and friendlier communities.

The realization that complex behaviors as well as the foundation upon which they are built—emotions and feelings—are really just expressions of genes and biochemistry molded by the environment can be unsettling to some. I've taught this for years and generally find that people with strong religious beliefs are more apt to disbelieve the science yet they aren't alone in their subjective acceptance when science questions existentialism. Secular and religious alike accept free will and for different reasons consider the biological basis of behaviors to be threatening, yet the science is no less sound than the theory of gravity. I'm often asked questions like, "What about complex emotions? What about love? Can the feelings I have for my baby or boyfriend or dog literally be boiled down to just genes and reactions?"

No, but they are simple and complex expressions of genes and biochemical reactions that are molded by environmental experiences. We all feel love, for example, and we all feel a sense of protection when our loved ones are threatened, but what really is "love"? Women with postpartum depression don't feel love for their newborn. In fact, the bond between mother and child slowly develops after birth and is a byproduct of endocrine actions requiring two hormones: prolactin and oxytocin. The bond develops more rapidly with nursing as stimulating the nipple also stimulates release of both hormones that then coordinate milk production and secretion as well as activate the neural regions necessary for forming attachments. Oxytocin also stimulates uterine contractions during orgasm. This dual functionality links the physical acts—having sex or nursing a child—to the emotional states and bond formation shared between partners and between mother and child. I'm oversimplifying of course, but not as much as you might think. Consider the tilapia.

This tofu of the sea is boring to eat and not particularly pretty. However, it is also incredibly fascinating. Tilapia live in both fresh and sea water and freely move between both. They thrive in the dirtiest of environments, waters that kill most fish, have been called the cockroach of the sea and can starve for months without losing weight. From a physiological perspective, they're superfish! They are also mouth brooders. After males fertilize eggs laid in a nest, the female carries the developing embryos in her mouth and even after the fry hatch and begin swimming, she continues to protect them in her mouth by signaling when threats approach. Does she "love" her babies? That's a philosophical discussion that can't be answered, but she definitely cares for them and has behavioral responses consistent with what we consider love in our species. Parental care, however, is completely eliminated by removing the anterior pituitary gland, which is where prolactin is produced, yet caregiving is restored with a simple prolactin injection. So is prolactin love? No, love is prolactin and oxytocin and serotonin and estradiol and testosterone and myriad other biochemical expressions that respond to environmental stimuli like gentle touches, candle-lit dinners and the sweet, sweet baritone of Barry White.

The biology of mammalian sex, literally every aspect of sexual development and function, gender identity, sexual orientation and emotional bonding, result from a developmental process. They cannot be defined by any one thing, whether it's genotypic sex and the presence or absence of the Y chromosome, gonadal sex and the presence of testes or ovaries or phenotypic sex described by genitalia and other sex-dependent anatomies. The differentiating process may start with a Y chromosome, but the process very often never starts or is interrupted or altered. It's also subject to the same genetic variabilities that make us all unique and this produces variability in the final outcome: variability in our genitalia, variability in menstrual cycles, variability in sperm production and quality and, yes, variability in gender identity and sexual orientation.

Problems in the process often occur and when discovered, they're managed by a pediatric endocrinologist whose favorite response to the pregnancy question "Do you want a boy or a girl?" is "yes." Such problems produce sexual ambiguities that make classifying the sex of newborns difficult to impossible as genotypic and phenotypic sex don't always match. For example, a genetic XY male could have female genitalia and fully developed breasts, as with androgen insensitivity syndrome, while a genetic XX female could have male genitalia and other masculine traits including massive musculature and facial hair due to adrenal hyperplasia. Because the process and hormones that control development of genitalia also cause female and male brains to structurally and functionally differ, people can have matching genotypic and phenotypic sex yet still develop gender dysphoria. To put it bluntly, the sex of their brain differs from that of their body. This is real. This is natural. This is not a choice.

Let me blow your mind just one last time before getting to my massively belabored point. Genotypic males with XY chromosomes have given birth to beautiful bouncing babies. It's true and it's rare, but it has happened several times with a little help from science and from compassionate pediatric endocrinologists like Dr. Claude Migeon, a former and famous colleague from the Johns Hopkins University School of Medicine.

Claude managed a patient with Swyer syndrome where the SRY gene transfers to the X chromosome. "SRY" is an acronym for sex-determining region of the Y chromosome and the SRY gene, which is also known as TDF or testis-determining factor, is the magical holy grail of sex determination. It starts the entire process of converting a bipotential gonad that is neither testicle nor ovary into the former. Without SRY, the default developmental program is female. If the SRY gene contains mutations or if it isn't induced to produce sufficient amounts of the SRY protein, the baby's sex can be difficult and sometimes impossible to define. If it's transferred to X chromosome, as with Swyer syndrome, the gonad never develops into an ovary or testicle, but everything else follows the default program for producing a healthy baby girl. *Presence of the Y chromosome is itself not the harbinger of all things male.*

Remember that the default developmental programming is female. This includes not only reproductive tissues but also brain and muscle and other tissues whose development are normally influenced by testosterone. It's also impossible to reverse the programming because the fetal tissues that would normally have been masculinized into the male reproductive anatomy are gone months before birth. Thus, this genetically XY "boy"—not my definition—was born with a vulva, vagina, uterus, fallopian tubes and feminized brain. Because she lacked ovaries, her parents consented to hormone replacement therapy that mimicked the normal pubertal changes and the genetically XY "boy" had a normal healthy childhood and adolescence as a normal healthy "girl"—my and the entire

Chapter 5

scientific community's definition. Why "girl"? Because sex results from a process, not a thing.

This amazing young woman excelled at scholastics and athletics and competed as an Ivy League Division I student athlete. Because it's pertinent to the discussion, I'll note that she was extremely beautiful and elegantly feminine. Helen of Troy would have been envious. She met her future husband in college and when they decided to have a family, she turned to Claude for advice. Her parents rightly or wrongly never fully explained her condition and forbade Claude from doing so, a handicap that thankfully no longer exists in Maryland's privacy laws. She understood she couldn't get pregnant, but she didn't know why.

Claude grew emotional at this point in the presentation. He was a model physician and person, with compassion and empathy for his patients, yet after years of treating her, attending her graduations and marriage and spending holiday celebrations with the family, he found himself for the first time an outsider, respected for his intellect and manner but no longer for comfort.

The miracle of birth came not from an immaculate conception but from medical professionals including endocrinologists and obstetricians with expertise in reproductive medicine and *in vitro* fertilization. Her sister donated eggs that were fertilized by her husband and subsequently implanted into her uterus, preconditioned for acceptance with progesterone therapy. God may have failed her, but science did not.

Now ask yourself. What defines sex? Is it genes or genitalia? What about the capacity to produce gametes, eggs and sperm or to give birth? It's definitely not sexual orientation, but could it be gender identity? The average pediatrician can't define it at birth nor can specialists like pediatric endocrinologists, at least not with absolute certainty.

Sex cannot be defined in binarity. The imposition of politicians to do so is incorrect, offensive and immoral, all at grand scales. Science can inform decisions to help govern the continuum of sexes, but only you can define your sex.

So here's my final question. Knowing what you now know, that sex isn't a result of a thing but a process, that natural variability controlling the process as well as problems in the process itself introduce ambiguities complicating attempts to define sex, should transgender athletes be allowed to compete against the cisgendered?

Claude's patient developed *in utero* and throughout childhood and adolescence in the absence of testosterone. The adrenal gland also produces "weak androgens," which are testosterone-like molecules, but her exposure was identical to every other cisgendered female. This is an important distinction because testosterone increases muscle protein synthesis, creating larger and stronger muscles. It stimulates proliferation of muscle satellite cells, the stem cells that repair muscle after strenuous exercise and contribute to exercise-induced changes in muscle mass and performance. It stimulates the release of other growth-promoting hormones and enhances the strength of elastic fibers and bones. It also enhances core metabolism, enabling athletes to work out longer and harder.

Some of the hormone's actions are actually mediated by its conversion to estradiol. This partially explains the pubertal changes to muscle and bone in girls, although estradiol, which is produced at far higher levels in girls than in boys, also directs changes in fat deposition that are unique to girls, changes that lower their center of gravity, increase their body fat percentage and cause hips and breasts to bulge. In fact, most girls actually become less athletic with puberty due to these changes and due to a widening pelvis that can alter running mechanics. Because puberty begins at an earlier age in girls, when the muscle to bone mass ratio is low, they also experience more hip and knee injuries during puberty. All of this produces a stark performance discrepancy between cisgendered sexes that is probably best illustrated in track. The women's all-time world records for 100m, 200m, 400m, 800m and mile, for example, aren't good enough to have won the boy's 2023 Maryland state championship for any of these events (see table 5.1). Maryland is a small state known more for lacrosse and basketball and definitely not for track so comparisons to larger states are even more enlightening. In California, only one world record holder would have even placed in the top 10.

Claude's patient exemplifies the problem of disqualifying athletes based solely on genotypic sex. She never experienced testosterone's virilizing effects and her successes stem solely from superior genetics,

CHAPTER 5

Table 5.1 World Record Finishes in Boys' State Championships

Event	Athlete	Time	Place in Maryland	Place in California
100m	Florence Griffith Joyner	10.49	3	18
200m	Florence Griffith Joyner	21.34	4	19
400m	Marita Koch	47.60	2	7
800m	Jarmila Kratochvílová	1:53.28	5	>25
mile	Sifan Hassan	4:12.33	2	11

hard work and dedication. Disqualifying her and athletes like her from competitions would be a travesty. It could also be financially devastating to the athlete who would be barred from scholarships, sponsorships and prizes and—politicians beware—to the disqualifying authorities that eventually lose the ensuing lawsuits. Male genotypic athletes who transition to female after puberty, however, clearly benefit from testosterone exposure and as I've explained, this includes much more than changes to muscle mass that despite some opinions will not fully or even significantly transition to a female state. What changes do occur will be gradual and such athletes will without doubt benefit greatly from puberty's virilization. Allowing them to compete against cisgendered females who have not benefited from this exposure is patently unfair, also without doubt.

So what should be done? Disqualifying trans athletes is clearly discriminatory and I'll add reprehensible. Those who transitioned after puberty may have an unfair athletic advantage, but the competitions could be easily structured to allow everyone to participate and to respect the physical and psychological needs of all youth athletes regardless of gender identity. This is the challenge that governing authorities should be considering rather than political agendas.

The solution is painfully obvious for individualized sports: just let them play. Trans athletes could compete among either cis athlete group but would be ranked only with other self-identifying trans athletes.

Having an unfair advantage is only concerning when the rewards are at stake, so segregate the ribbons, medals and trophies but not the athletes. This is done for disabled athletes and there's no excuse for not applying the same standard. It's also being done with the Boston, New York and Chicago marathons and other road races. In fact, the Road Runners Club of America has officially adopted transgender/non-binary divisions using a publicly available guide (https://nonbinaryrunning.com/) produced by Jake Fedorowski, an activist for transgender/non-binary rights and a competitive runner. USA Triathlon has also adopted transgender/non-binary divisions, setting precedent for the USATF and other governing bodies of individual sports.

Finding equality for team sports is only slightly more difficult. Safety should be the primary concern, although I suspect the six-foot, ten-inch, 240-pound female-transitioning power forward is a rarity and in the unlikely event that this individual and her family would rather play against cisgendered girls who are vastly inferior in talent, which would never happen, a simple safety clause in a school district's charter could be used to justify such athletes playing with their competitive peers: male cisgender athletes. This scenario would allow most trans athletes to compete among their social peers and a very few to compete among their competitive peers. I suspect this latter solution will be unacceptable to a small percentage of politicians on both sides of the aisle and to the 24-hour viewers of Fox News and MSNBC, although I also suspect the pragmatic among us and the vast majority of parents reading this are currently applauding.

Anyone worried that an unscrupulous trans athlete would sneak their way to a championship should realize that incognito participation is already happening. It's astronomically rare, mind you, and it should be noted that they're probably not sneaking but are either unaware of their genotypic sex or are only interested in getting that participation trophy. How rare? A recent study linked and referenced here suggests that roughly 300,000 US children ages 13 to 17, only 1.4%, identify as transgender.[1] The percentage drops to 0.5% for adults ages 25 to 64, possibly reflecting the natural uncertainty and confusion over gender identity and sexual orientation. The Aspen Institute's National Survey of

Children's Health indicates that 56.1% of children ages 6 to 17 participate in organized sports, but the number decreases with age and those regularly playing at the competitive levels being debated are only 41.7%. The Trevor Project, a non-profit organization to prevent suicide among LGBTQ children that also conducts mental health research, reports that only 17% of transgender children ages 13 to 18 participate in some kind of sport, not organized or competitive sports per se. If we apply the same attrition rate from the Aspen Institute's study to the Trevor Project's estimates, the country is falling apart because less than 0.2% of its children just want to play.

Note that 0.2% is most definitely an overestimate. Gender identity isn't malleable and can't be consciously changed like shoes or political party affiliations. The fact that only 0.5% of adults identify as transgender suggests that the real percentage of competitive transgender youth athletes is 2.8 times lower or 0.07%. This equates to roughly 15,000 kids nationwide. Kids! Kids who want to run for PRs, celebrate with their team and grow as adults. Kids who like all others want a safe environment to just feel normal.

Meilani's Take (18 Years Old)

The person I remember most from my first day of school in Maryland was Andrea Ye. I had arrived from Idaho only a couple weeks earlier and she bravely invited the new girl to join her in a crowded elementary school lunchroom. She was unapologetically welcoming, kind and although the conversation flowed, she seemed more nervous than I was. I quickly realized that we were fundamentally different people as even then I was extraverted with a bit type A, comfortable in a spotlight, whereas she was reserved and shy. We were cordial yet clearly incompatible and because my eventual friend group would rarely interact with hers, I began noticing her less and less. It wasn't until the following year when she changed her name to Beluga Whale when she took her first step into the spotlight.

Our teachers instructed us to use her new name and to accept her new masculine appearance. Her feminine light pink tops were replaced with baggy boys' tees and her hair was styled in a short pixie cut. She seemed content and confident when sitting alone at her desk but would quickly turn away from eye contact and timidly stare at her feet when walking the halls. No explanation was provided for her stark new look or new name.

While I can understand the need to transition and respect her belief in a process, the choice to identify as an animal, much less a whale, was in my opinion a horrible mistake. It fueled the middle school gossip and the avalanche of inevitable teasing and bullying. Girls whispered and giggled behind her back and the popular boys openly taunted her, yelling, "Here comes the whale" as she walked past. They'd parade her around like a circus act, mocking her name and pretending to swim with her. What I found most confusing, however, was that she never protested. In fact, she smiled and laughed at the spectacle, at herself, as the hazing worsened. I could never tell if she recognized or was oblivious to the maliciousness and patronization and I couldn't imagine how anyone could endure it or why teachers allowed it. This was almost a daily occurrence until one day when it wasn't. She suddenly stopped coming to school and I honestly don't remember when or even being surprised. You can imagine my shock, however, when *he* returned as Alex Ye during a high school Zoom class.

Most of my classmates didn't recognize him at first. There were no gasps or laughs though, just comments whispered between friends in their respective circles. He, Alex, also seemed much more at peace with himself, confident even, volunteering in class or to participate in groups. Looks can be deceiving though because later that semester, he was removed from school for disclosing "homicidal ideation" and arrested for threats of mass violence. In what the press described as a "manifesto," he outlined plans to shoot up our high school and the neighboring elementary school, citing revenge for past bullying in what he described was a "memoir."

I will never understand the mental and physical challenges that Alex and other transgender people experience before, during or after their transition. Not to mention the additional obstacles society forces upon them. I would also never suggest that transgender people are more violent than cisgendered as I suspect the exact opposite is probably true. In fact, I'd be astonished if it wasn't. The example instead emphasizes the tragic nature of anyone experiencing gender dysphoria as Alex's story is one of a tragedy experienced and a tragedy avoided. It illustrates the desperation of a traumatized child and the need for empathy over ridicule. I empathize with the Alex that I knew and with transgender athletes, their need to fit in and the desire to compete. Nevertheless, I also recognize that high-level competition is restricted by limits in roster size, scholarships, awards and records. This in turn means that transgender inclusion at this level comes at a direct cost to cisgendered athletes.

Demonstrating empathy and ensuring equal opportunity for all athletes is a must. Transgender athletes deserve the opportunity to compete, in some way and in some venue, but not if it's based on an unfair advantage over cisgender or even other transgender athletes. The NCAA Transgender Student-Athlete Participation Policy attempts to identify and disqualify unfair advantage by screening testosterone levels at three different points: before any regular season competition, before the first NCAA Championship event and before any competition in the non-championship segment. It's informed by scientific guidelines, but it assumes the presence or absence of testosterone alone is *the* determinant for advantage. It ignores the fact that muscles, bones, tendons, ligaments—the entire body—developed in the presence of testosterone and that blocking the hormone well after puberty diminishes but does not eliminate these effects.

I can't imagine being able to distinguish a transgender women who transitioned before puberty from a cisgendered woman. Their development wouldn't have been affected by male reproductive hormones so the transgender inclusion debate really centers on children who transition after puberty. The best and probably most famous example is Lia Thomas. She was a transgender female swimmer at the University of Pennsylvania who transitioned from the men's to women's team and from obscurity to notoriety. She smashed women's records, won a national championship and sparked controversy on her team, campus and eventually in Congress, all while transitioning in the middle of her collegiate career.

Her case was heavily publicized as were her teammates' opposition, most notably from Paula Scanlan who perfectly describes the issues in testimony to Congress and in a letter to the university newspaper.[2] She and other female athletes and coaches have since written and spoken extensively on the subject.[3] People like Riley Gaines (swimming, University of Kentucky), Sia Liilii (volleyball, University of Nevada), Brooke Slusser (co-captain volleyball, San Jose State University) and Melissa Batie-Smoose (associate coach volleyball, San Jose State University) as well as the LGBTQ+ activist and professional tennis great Martina Navratilova universally agree that transgender female athletes should not be allowed to compete against cisgendered athletes when the competitive advantage is evident. They readily express sympathy and respect for transgender female athletes and recognize their right to compete, again in some way and in some venue, but not at the expense of cisgendered rights and safety.

Ms. Thomas was eventually banned from professional swimming by its governing body, World Aquatics, whose official policy only allows transgender female athletes to compete if they "have not experienced any part of male puberty beyond Tanner Stage 2 (of puberty) or before age 12, whichever is later." This policy also applies to collegiate transgender female swimmers because Phase 1 of the NCAA Transgender Student-Athlete Participation Policy defers to sport governing bodies.[4] Phase 2 is the testosterone screening mentioned earlier, which ends the debate for swimming but not for other collegiate sports that lack similar governing bodies or policies.

The NCAA president Charlie Baker testified in Congress that less than 10 out of approximately 510,000 collegiate athletes identify as trans, just 0.002%. Other than isolated examples, does this policy or issue really have an actual impact? NCAA policies don't regulate school, club, travel or recreational leagues. To this, my father suggests creating a "league of their own" where transgender athletes can compete with cisgender athletes in some individual sports like track or swimming with separate awards and records for each group. While this demonstrates empathy and provides equal opportunity to transgender athletes, it also risks ostracizing them in what I consider to be an imperfect compromise.

Including transgender girls and women in team sports can present and has presented safety concerns. Bruises and sprains are common on the field, but not the fractures, tears and concussions that often occur when playing against opponents who are significantly bigger, stronger and faster. This concern applies not only to team sports with mix-gendered athletes but also to games between small and large communities. I've had multiple injuries, some serious, some very serious and some requiring surgery followed by months of physical therapy and almost all resulted from collisions with girls not much bigger than I am. This is in addition to the broken arms and legs and an insurmountable number of concussions I've seen happen during my own soccer games. Imagine the carnage of introducing stronger and faster players several inches taller and 100 pounds heavier than I am, my brother for example or boys from my high school soccer team. Am I willing to risk a broken arm or would I be looking to change my sport?

As my father suggests, safety clauses in school or league charters could allow trans- and cisgendered girls and women to play together in team sports. I like to think of this as "like-bodied leagues" where most trans athletes seeking social interactions would compete among their social peers and a very few to compete among their competitive peers. This may again be an imperfect compromise, but it provides equal, although I admit not identical, opportunity while maintaining a safe playing environment.

Chapter 6

Bowling Balls, Meat Cleavers and Chainsaws

I once saw a comedian juggle a bowling ball, meat cleaver and chainsaw. To prove the authenticity of the cleaver, he used a wooden stool as a cutting board and sliced a tomato in half, saying without any emotion, "Razor. Sharp. Cleaver." He next dropped the bowling ball onto a tomato half saying, "Razor. Sharp. Bowling ball," and then proceeded to demolish the stool with the chainsaw. When finished, he calmly turned off the chainsaw, lowered it to the stage, removed his safety goggles and slowly turned toward the audience with an uncomfortable, almost psychotic smile. Andy Kauffman would have loved the act.

Watching him juggle all three items was both awe inspiring and mesmerizing. You imagined the difficulty of balancing the vastly different weights and handholds. Catching the bowling ball in his palm, the cleaver and chainsaws by their differently molded handles, each spinning wildly in the air while the engine of the chainsaw roared. You could see the sweat beading on his forehead and when the act ended, I felt sweat running down the middle of my back: nervousness by proxy!

It was a thoroughly entertaining act. The comedian never stopped cracking jokes until the finale when he caught and threw the cleaver to the floor, impaling the stage and picking up the remains of the tomato. He then caught the chainsaw in the other hand, smashed the tomato on his forehead and snatched the bowling ball, which pulled him into a bow. The audience exploded, pandemonium ensued and the comedian gleefully exited stage right.

I'm sure the comedian practiced incessantly, initially mastering the juggling in step-wise fashion, possibly starting with the cleaver and chainsaw because they both had handles and then combined the bowling ball with either one before juggling all three. I suspect he designed safeguards to protect himself and the audience before finally honing his punchlines. I also suspect that despite his best efforts and total commitment to his art, he made an occasional mistake. Think about that for a moment. What would happen if, for example, he dropped the tomato and it rolled off the stage? Would the act still be entertaining? Probably, but what if the cleaver impaled his foot or even worse, the spinning chainsaw was hurled into the audience, decapitating a lovely couple on their first date?

Coaches aren't comedians and coaches don't hurl deadly objects into unexpecting crowds, but they do juggle. They juggle the multiple interests of players, parents and leagues. They juggle to develop skills, mental preparedness and motivation. They juggle winning, losing and sportsmanship. The multi-tasking skillset required of a good coach is unrivaled in my opinion, which explains why so many coaches struggle with the juggle.

The primary responsibilities of any coach, at any level and for any sport, are to teach, mentor and manage: the Holy Trinity of coaching. Mastering each requires different skills, different emotional commitments and different degrees of knowledge and although nobody gets killed if mentoring is hurled into the third row, the results of dropping any one of the three primary responsibilities can be frustrating at best and truly disastrous at worst.

If you've had any experience with organized coaching, either as an athlete or maybe as a parent, sibling or friend of an athlete or even as a spectator or fan, you've probably witnessed the frustration and maybe even a disaster. Simple mistakes, say a dropped ball or baton, a missed goal or forgetting to play or do as instructed, can have what seems to be monumental consequences. I contest, however, that these are actually inconsequential to the bigger picture, to the frustration that results from repeated mistakes, for example, or to the abuse, depression and even violence that can and has occurred when the Holy Trinity is ignored.

I learned to teach as a graduate student. Unlike humanities, art and liberal art programs, my particular program and most scientific fields didn't include formal training in pedagogy, the science of teaching. Instead, graduate students were required to teach for at least a full year and were metaphorically tossed into the deep end of the pool, serving as teaching assistants or "TAs" where they led discussions or laboratory exercises. Most struggled to keep their head above water, thrashing their limbs violently as they raced to stay a chapter ahead of their students and although all TAs are managed by one or more professors, very few are provided a structured pedagogical program beyond weekly TA meetings to cover grading assignments or to practice laboratory exercises. The art of actually teaching, in my experience as a TA and as a professor, was never addressed. Not surprisingly, most TAs dislike the experience and are ecstatic when their tour of duty ends. Research is rightly their top priority, not teaching, as master's and PhD degrees are generally awarded for the creation of knowledge not its dissemination. Yet everyone who has ever taught or was trained to teach, whether they were good, bad or mediocre at it, literally everyone has the same impression: teaching is hard and teaching well is extremely difficult.

Mentoring is often confused with teaching as they generally occur in similar settings and because mentoring requires teaching. The opposite, however, isn't the case as teaching can occur without any mentoring altogether, say in a very large classroom or on a professional sports team where specialized coaches teach specialized tasks and mentoring either occurs organically or is championed by the head coach alone. Differences in teaching and mentoring are often described in scale, by relationships and duties, all of which are true, yet the key difference is legacy. Teachers instill knowledge and test comprehension, mentors provide a path for using knowledge and a safe environment to fail. Teachers eventually stop teaching, as when class ends or students graduate, but a mentor's role continuously evolves and morphs as pupils develop, often succeeding or failing in ways that mirror those of the mentor. A good mentor's role ends when the casket is lowered or the flame is lit and can be traced through a familial pedigree, a phylogeny actually where direct descendants evolve as orthologs and paralogs appear almost at random as mentoring styles are emulated.

I was a natural. The act of communicating what I knew and "how to do" was innate and as a result, learning to teach was difficult but not arduous. It helped that I had excellent mentors—see how it works—all who served by example and some who took more active roles. When I was an undergraduate, I lived on Gilligan's Island, literally, the island in Kaneohe Bay where the introduction to the iconic 1970s sitcom was filmed. The island was and still is home to the Hawai'i Institute of Marine Biology, a premier institute with premier faculty who liked working late into the evening. My rent was paid with shuttle duties, driving scientists on and off the island in tiny unstable skiffs at all hours of the night. I roomed with my TAs, I worked for my professors, I lived and breathed marine biology and I was surrounded by science nerds craving the attention of wanting students. It. Was. Awesome!

I immersed myself in the science. I emulated my roommates Bill Tyler and John Godwin as well as my professor and lab director, Gordon Grau, all superb teachers of science. I know their names mean nothing to the reader, but they mean the world to me because the sincerity and objectivity of their advice, critiques and opinions were and still are highly valued; that's how mentorship works. When I went to Berkeley for my graduate studies, I worked for quite possibly the two best life science instructors at Cal, Professors Karl Nicoll and Gary Firestone, both superb orators with an uncanny ability to make personal connections in crowds of students. Later in my academic career, I met Professor Bob Goldberg while I was on sabbatical at UCLA. Bob had won multiple teaching awards and shared my enthusiasm for teaching. He was also a model mentor and as such invited me to lectures and coffee breaks where we'd discuss how best to structure a learning environment, overcoming the challenges of teaching large diverse audiences, the benefits of real-time engagement and techniques for motivating students without scaring the crap out of them. When I moved to Washington State, I met Professor Phil Senger who in my mind was undeniably the best teacher I ever met, the best of the best. Phil taught me the importance of building trust and respect with your students, that fear and intimidation were your enemies and that students appreciated humility as long as you recognized and addressed your shortcomings. Empathy, however, was the most important trait. Indeed, all of my teaching mentors emphasized the importance of walking in your students' shoes, remembering the feeling of test anxiety and performance stress and multi-tasking the scholastic, social, work and sometimes athletic demands of a student. Like I said, teaching is hard.

Now close your eyes. Imagine the coaches from your past or the youth coaches in your life. Remember how they talked to you and your kids, how they behaved in practice and on the sideline. Did they project trust and respect or did they rule with fear? Were they reassuring or intimidating? Did they demonstrate humility with a willingness to admit and correct their faults or did they deflect criticisms and questions with excuses? Were they empathetic, understanding your or your child's diversity of challenges and anxieties, or were they dismissive?

Were they coaching for you or your kids or were they coaching for themselves?

Memories of my childhood coaches are mostly negative, some even terrifying. My high school football coach would hit kids on the helmet with a golf club. My high school wrestling coach broke a teammate's back with an illegal move, permanently crippling the kid. My high school baseball coach knew little of the sport and basically played the popular kids regardless of skill or lack thereof and my high school track coach didn't exist. I was a distance runner and our only coach worked with sprinters while the distance kids mostly just jogged around town. One of my youth baseball coaches, by contrast, was one of the better coaches I've ever met: Bob Freeman, a former minor league player in the Cincinnati Reds farm system. Bob never made it to the majors and, as far as I know, never made it beyond the Rookie or Single A levels. He was short and stout, not particularly strong and bore a strong resemblance to a mustachioed Pillsbury Doughboy. Nevertheless, his command of fundamental skills was enough to impress and he was wickedly accurate with a fungo bat, a long thin baseball bat coaches use to hit balls during practice. In between a blue-collar retail job and coaching youth baseball, Bob still worked as a scout for the Reds, a secret he carefully guarded to protect his objectivity as well as to ward off the well-meaning lobbyist, a parent or coach who despite good intentions had literally no nose for talent.

Bob was good people. One of the nicest, most sincere and truly caring people that I've ever met. We developed a close relationship over the years that lasted well past my high school days and I admit to feeling guilty for not maintaining a connection after I moved away. In many ways, my teaching and coaching style resemble his, which was based on a hierarchal structure that develops and then reinforces the fundamental physical skills of the game before developing the mental skills or *baseball IQ*. "Fundamentals and brains," he'd say, "are all that's needed to be a good baseball player." Throwing with accuracy was prioritized over throwing hard. Consistency, not flash, was considered key to being a good defensive player. Whether a batter got on base by a hit, walk, error or hit-by-pitch was inconsequential to Bob. The goal was to reach first base and to move runners, period. Bob truly was ahead of his time, as anyone familiar with the game of baseball or who has ever seen the movie *Moneyball* would attest.

The value of Bob's focus on physical and mental preparedness, on emphasizing basic skills and intelligent play, was evident in his success. Bob almost always won the town championship including the three years I played for him. He would regularly beat travel all-star teams from much larger towns and it didn't matter whether he coached with an assistant or by himself. It also didn't matter who played for him because the championship team had the last pick in the following year's little league draft. When I asked if his scouting skills enabled him to stack the team during the draft he said, "Yes, but I draft for coachability, not skill."

I believe Bob was also a good if not great mentor. This comes primarily from hindsight as I admit we never discussed mentoring directly. We did, however, discuss playing with intelligence, shutting out distractions, leaving mistakes in the dugout and owning my accomplishments as well as my failures, all of which left this undersized skinny late bloomer with a gargantuan nose and braces beaming with confidence. I also witnessed Bob mentor troubled teens. Kids from poor or broken families who wore hand-me-downs that never fit. Kids with facial bruises that mysteriously appeared. Kids with anger issues who themselves were both bullied and bullies. One in particular was being raised by his two older siblings, a brother still in high school and a sister who lived in a different town and who seldom visited. Dad was an invalid, never fully recovering from a stroke, and Mom just disappeared one day. Some of these kids had talent, most didn't, but they all carried the shame of abandonment, poverty or abuse. Baseball was a carrot in their lives, maybe not *the* carrot, but a positive influence and source of pride and accomplishment in an unnecessarily stressful and sometimes painful existence.

It's important to understand that this community wasn't an exception but the norm. It was and is an agricultural community filled with good hardworking people who love their families, schools and sports but often lacked the financial resources to properly support all of the above. The same could be said of many inner-city neighborhoods or mining towns or the entire state of West Virginia. Coaches were usually dads spending time with their kids. Dads who cared for the kids as much as their communities yet, to be honest, hadn't a clue how to coach. One could never fault their motivation, only their approach.

I personally have bigger issues with professional youth coaches than with the well-meaning mom or dad. The former most likely never received formal training during their semi-successful athletic career that in a twisted reality substitutes for coaching credentials—*doing* is most definitely not the same as *coaching*—and although parent coaches are even less likely to have been formally trained, nobody expects them to be any good. They shouldn't be abusive, of course, or create an unsafe learning environment, but only the most misguided, deranged or unstable among us would seriously criticize a parent's coaching abilities. We're thankful for their commitment, we complain about playing time and in the end, we accept the situation for what it is, a nice opportunity to exercise, socialize and celebrate. Professionals, on the other hand, are rightfully held to a higher standard yet few are formally trained and even fewer, in my experience, embrace or even understand the Holy Trinity.

So what should we expect of our coaches? Winning? Hopefully not, although some degree of competitiveness is expected at all levels of organized play and should be structured into the learning environment.

CHAPTER 6

I assume most parents and child athletes would also expect the degree of competitiveness to increase as athletes matriculate into more organized play, as when transitioning from backyard games to recreational leagues and especially into travel and even elite leagues. Everyone would agree that safety should be the top priority regardless of league status or competitive level, but that's about where the consensus ends. How should health, fitness and conditioning be balanced with skills development? How are strategy and teamwork balanced with the equitable exposure of individual athletes? Everyone wants to win, but at what cost and who decides? Do coaches make these decisions in a vacuum or are they governed by league managers? If the latter, is there oversight? Do we as parents and athletes have any say in the matter? Of course we should, although in my experience as an athlete, however poor, and as a coach and parent of two youth athletes, our influence is generally limited to playing the game and writing checks, respectively. This is fine when team and coaching priorities are well articulated, but what if they're not? What if they're not even established? Asking questions is helpful as is digging on the internet, but the information is often superficial, especially regarding oversight. How are we even to know what questions to ask?

Enter the Aspen Institute.[1] This international non-profit, non-partisan and non-government research institute (aka think tank) was founded in 1949 with the goal to "foster leadership based on enduring values and to provide a nonpartisan venue for dealing with critical issues," one of which is youth sports and coaching. It defines itself as "an educational and policy studies organization" with what I perceive as a mixed mission of discovery and dissemination. Think of it as a vertically integrated one-stop shop for creating and spreading knowledge to a mass/lay audience, something I wish all institutes of higher education would but almost never do.

Core areas of study include business and society, energy and environment, justice and civic identity as well as health and sport plus five other areas, each divided into several separate programs of focus. Health and sport, for example, includes the Sports and Society Program that studies the future of sports and holds conferences or summits to explore how sports, athletics and exercise intersect with different aspects of our society and culture. Project Play is particularly relevant and has produced numerous publications assessing youth sports in general as well as school sports. Project Play also works with targeted municipalities and leaders to improve child access to sports and to build healthy communities. I encourage everyone interested in youth sports to immerse themselves in the Aspen Institute website, which is a goldmine of information for coaches, school and district athletic directors, league administrators, and especially parents.

A cornerstone of Project Play is the Children's Bill of Rights in Sports, developed collaboratively by a drafting committee composed of nine directors or C-level leaders from Project Play itself as well as Athletes for Hope, the Center for Sport and the Law at the University of Baltimore School of Law, the Centre for Sport and Human Rights, the US Center for SafeSport and other non-profit human rights organizations. The bill is presented as a collection of "guardrails," although a more apt description in my opinion would be "foundations." Guardrails prevent misdirection but not design failures and are by definition limited in scope and impact. They protect cars from soaring off a cliff but not the underlying brake failure that caused the accident. My point shouldn't be lost in semantics as the cornerstone of the cornerstone, the primary reason the bill was written in the first place, was to prevent abuse and injury and to ensure a safe, equitable and quality playing experience, which is impossible unless engineered into the athletic experience from its inception.

The bill is logical and sensical. It is also carefully crafted for a child's physical and mental health needs that naturally differ from those of adults. It recognizes that children require nurturing, safe and distraction-free environments to play. It protects their access and freedom to play, it empowers their voice and it guarantees a quality playing experience. Note how little is focused on the actual teaching or managing of play, just half of the third right, and how much is devoted to mentoring and safety, which recognizes the uniqueness of coaching children. The Holy Trinity is indeed reflected in the bill, albeit disproportionately.

Chapter 6

Children's Bill of Rights in Sports[2]
1. *To play sports.*
   Organizations should make every effort to accommodate children's interests to participate, and to help them play with peers from diverse backgrounds.
2. *To safe and healthy environments.*
   Children have the right to play in settings free from all forms of abuse (physical, emotional, sexual), hazing, violence, and neglect.
3. *To qualified program leaders.*
   Children have the right to play under the care of coaches and other adults who pass background checks and are trained in key competencies.
4. *To developmentally appropriate play.*
   Children have a right to play at a level commensurate with their physical, mental and emotional maturity, and their emerging athletic ability. They should be treated as young people first, athletes second.
5. *To share in the planning and delivery of their activities.*
   Children have the right to share their viewpoints with coaches and for their insights to be incorporated into activities.
6. *To an equal opportunity for personal growth.*
   Programs should invest equally in all child athletes, free of discrimination based on any personal or family characteristic.
7. *To be treated with dignity.*
   Children have the right to participate in environments that promote the values of sportsmanship, of respect for opponents, officials, and the game.
8. *To enjoy themselves.*
   Children have the right to participate in activities they consider fun, and which foster the development of friendships and social bonds.

Universal adoption of the bill has the potential to transform youth sports programs. Entire leagues and conferences could be engineered from the ground up to address inequalities, to safeguard from abuses, to ensure fairness in play and instruction and to protect. Imagine a system where coaches, team managers and league/conference administrators were evaluated on performance standards according to each right rather than on wins and losses. Imagine the impact such changes could have on the quality of play and on managing the expectations of parents and players. All athletes perform better when stress is removed from the equation; when focus and concentration is limited to the field of play; when pressures to perform build from within and not from a belligerent fan, coach or parent; when teammates respect and trust one another; when expectations are grounded in objectivity and not favoritism and when players simply have fun, quite possibly the best motivator of all. Chemistry, cohesiveness, confidence, you name it, the bill is a means to all and to producing better and healthier athletes as well as to a more entertaining and enjoyable youth sports experience.

The bill is endorsed by professional and amateur athletic organizations like the NBA, PGA, NWSL, USA Baseball, USA Football, US Track and Field, US Olympic and Paralympic committees, Little League and many others. It is also endorsed by business and media outlets like Under Armour, Dick's Sporting Goods, ESPN and TeamSnap; by public health organizations like the American College of Sports Medicine and UNICEF; by several university/educational institutions like the Utah State University Families in Sport Lab and the University of Washington Center for Leadership in Athletics as well as by community recreation organizations like the YMCA, National Recreation and Parks Association and Girls on the Run, all to name just a few.

Considering how well the bill is endorsed, I was surprised to learn that none of my children's six high school coaches or their athletic director have ever heard of it. I consulted some of their former club coaches for baseball, soccer and track and none of them were familiar with the bill either. Some suggested their organizations had incorporated similar talking points into mission statements, although based on my family's experiences I have little confidence that such points ever seriously influenced how these organizations and their teams were managed and coached. Bullying by teammates and even coaches was common and even the school teams were more likely to be babysat than coached. One might expect superior coaching and an adherence to professionalism on advanced and elite travel clubs. After all, you get what you pay for, right? One would also expect a more challenging playing environment with highly skilled athletes and rigorous competition. All of this was true.

However, it was also true that mentorship was ignored as were most of the rights expressed earlier.

Were our coaches qualified? Did they embrace the Holy Trinity or its spirit? Most but not all understood the sport, some very well and some not so much. All of them taught aspects of the game and critical skills, all of them managed play during practice and in games and all of them organized the events. Very few, however, mentored the players and some were averse to the basic principle of coaching off the field or managing anything beyond strategy and skills: pure X-and-O types with "Just win baby!" mentalities. Were these latter coaches partially qualified or unqualified? Many if not most of the national athletic organizations endorsing the bill have formal certification programs and the bill is endorsed by only a fraction of the organizations available. Training opportunities are, therefore, abundant, which raises two very important questions: How well trained is the average coach and how well do they adhere to the philosophies and principals of the Holy Trinity?

Both questions are being answered in a collaborative venture—the first ever National Coach Survey—that grew out of the LiFE*sports* "positive youth development" program at Ohio State University.[3] "LiFE" is an acronym for Learning in Fitness and Education. The program uniquely applies the academic/extension mission of a typical land grant university toward youth athletics by conducting research, teaching future coaches and addressing the needs of Ohio's youth athletes and their communities. The program is small, composed of just 10 faculty and staff with about the same number of undergraduate and graduate students, yet its current and future impact far outweighs its size. LiFE*sports* is financed with "soft" money in the form of grants, donations and sponsorships from the likes of Nike, Project Play and the Susan Crown Exchange,[4] a non-profit foundation for child development and advocacy, all of which participated in the collaboration. Professor Dawn Anderson-Butcher and Assistant Professor Samantha Bates led the study and ultimately authored the final report that is free and publicly available.[5]

The study relied upon self-reported data, meaning that coaches were trusted at their word. Validity of such studies is notoriously difficult to assess, although surveyors are adept at detecting "response bias," an academic term for conscious and unconscious lying, with carefully structured surveys and questions and with rigorous statistical modeling. Topics included coaching histories, confidence in coaching skills, coaching philosophies and priorities, preparation and competencies working with specific populations and others. Data were then compared to each coach's perceived effectiveness, impact and self-reported winning percentage.

As expected, a supermajority of coaches expressed confidence in teaching athletic skills and tactics, two-thirds of the Holy Trinity, although possibly not as high as you might presume at 67%. Confidence waned significantly when coaches were asked about the intangible benefits of sports, one-third of the Holy Trinity and most of the bill, as only 29% expressed confidence in developing leaders and only 18% in adequately addressing unique mental health demands. In fact, about half of respondents felt prepared to manage intellectual, developmental or physical disabilities in general and 43% admitted to feeling unprepared to deal with common behavior problems like ADHD. Coaches with an education background and who were also school teachers were slightly more confident than non-educators in teaching life skills through sport, 52% versus 45%, which I find a bit disconcerting; professional teachers were only 7% more confident at teaching life skills, something they do every day, than those with no formal teacher training. Someone's overconfident and it certainly isn't the teachers!

The survey also found that schools are increasingly hiring coaches without education backgrounds as only 50% used teachers. This means that the vast majority of youth sports coaches—in school, recreational, travel, church and social clubs—will lack formal training in teaching and child development yet they're expected to teach and develop our children, many of whom might have behavior problems and/or a disability that coaches feel they can't confidently address. Moreover, community and unpaid coaches were "far less likely" to be evaluated or to have received formal training of any kind. A major finding of the study was that training matters. In fact, 91% of coaches with formal training report having a significant impact on creating role models and leaders whereas coaches without formal training report only 77%. Educators are properly positioned to witness and even document such successes as they see who leads in school and who's accepted to elite universities and programs. In general, they are also more involved in different aspects of a student athlete's life, which again questions the confidence of coaches who lack formal training. Maybe you think sports and life are mutually exclusive, that coaches should coach, teachers should teach and parents should parent. Fine, but a major finding of the survey is that coaches who prioritize life skills and mentoring report higher winning percentages.

Formal training clearly improves the athletic experience as well as the athlete, yet only 56% of respondents reported having obtained formal coaching credentials in the form of a certificate or license. Of these individuals, 12% describe their credentials as "not effective or slightly effective," 21% describe them as "somewhat effective" and 67% describe them as "moderately or extremely effective." If you assume no sampling bias in the survey, which most definitely is not the case, then only 37.5% of coaches (67% of the 56%) have received formal training with an official credentialing procedure that they themselves define as at least "moderately effective." This also means that 62.5% of coaches have never received any formal training that they'd define as being at best "somewhat effective."

Ask yourself, do you really trust your children learning anything in an environment where 62.5% of the teachers don't think they've received quality training? We might not care if it's a free class in beginner basket weaving, but what about activities with potential risks for serious or even fatal injury? Even with safeguards in place, do you want to pay for skills development without assurances that the teacher actually knows what and how skills should be developed?

I wasn't coaching when the survey was conducted and didn't participate. My daughter's high school soccer, cross-country, indoor and outdoor track coaches and their athletic director also didn't participate. In fact, they've never heard of the survey, of Project Play or even the Aspen Institute. A total of 10,485 coaches from throughout the country did participate, however, and the demographics of respondents were as you might have guessed: overwhelmingly white, male and middle aged. Coaches were recruited from different sports organizations, especially US

Youth Soccer, the US Soccer Federation and the US Soccer Foundation, from Washington and Ohio state high school athletic associations, from the Amateur Athletic Union (AAU) and from Little League. Soccer was disproportionately represented with 24% of respondents followed by baseball and basketball with 15% and 12%, respectively, and the remaining 49% from 36 other sports. 71% of coaches had at least a bachelor's degree, although only 20% of these were in sports- or education-related fields while 16% were in psychology.

To say that the survey is an undersampling is an understatement. Actually, I'd say it's a gross understatement, unless you think the vast majority of youth sports coaches are college-educated middle-aged white male soccer coaches with very little formal training in coaching and who live predominately in rural and suburban areas. Does this reflect the demographics in your area? Maybe, maybe not, although I suspect "white, male" and "little formal training" is fairly accurate for most.

The survey clearly represents only a fraction of the nation's coaches despite being the largest survey of coaches in our nation's history. It is in my scientific opinion an excellent starting point, a detailed preliminary assessment. It asks the right questions in the right way and it doesn't exaggerate conclusions that are purely descriptive and appropriately tempered. Drs. Anderson-Butcher and Bates recognize and discuss the study's limitations, primarily the overrepresentation of white male coaches as well as some statistical risks that for the fellow science geek out there are described as potential "type 1 errors." For the non-geeks, the survey reflects a genuine interest by the authors and the benefactors in bettering community health and improving every aspect of youth sports. Such accolades can't be said of the coaches, however, as survey data suggest that honesty was a problem for some if not many of them.

Coaches were asked to rank their coaching philosophies. The goal was to quantifiably assess their values and priorities based upon a list of 17 philosophies. Their most and least valued philosophies were then identified as the top or bottom 3, respectively. I've replotted the cumulative data in table 6.1 and added my own subjective categories for each philosophy based upon the Holy Trinity.

Table 6.1 Coaching Philosophy Rankings

Coaching Philosophies	Holy Trinity Category	Top 3	Bottom 3
Making sure all athletes play	Managing	29%	30%
Supporting athletes in being healthy and fit	Teaching	29%	9%
Helping athletes learn new sport-specific skills	Teaching	28%	13%
Helping athletes learn new life skills	Mentoring	35%	10%
Creating a sense of belonging through sport	Mentoring	29%	9%
Winning games or competitions	Managing	6%	62%
Teaching athletes to set their own goals and work toward them	Mentoring	23%	13%
Creating opportunities for athletes to learn from their mistakes	Teaching	12%	16%
Making sure athletes have fun	Mentoring	35%	13%
Teaching the love of sport	Teaching	29%	19%
Teaching athletes how to play fair	Mentoring	6%	35%
Ensuring athletes develop good sportspersonship	Mentoring	16%	24%
Creating a safe environment to prevent injuries	Managing	23%	33%

Note: The "Holy Trinity Category" was not part of the survey. *Source*: Anderson-Butcher, D. & Bates, S. (2022). National Coach Survey: Final Report. The Ohio State University LiFEsports Initiative, Columbus, OH. https://www.aspeninstitute.org/wp-content/uploads/2022/11/national-coach-survey-report-preliminary-analysis.pdf

"Helping athletes learn new life skills" and "Making sure athletes have fun" were the most popular, each appearing as a top 3 philosophy for 35% of coaches and a bottom 3 for 10% and 13%, respectively. Tied for third most popular was "Creating a sense of belonging through sport," which was a top 3 for 29% of coaches and a bottom 3 for 9%. This suggests that a little over one-third prioritize key aspects of sports mentoring as a top philosophy. Fair enough, although other mentoring philosophies were hardly valued at all like "Teaching athletes how to play fair" and "Ensuring athletes develop good sportspersonship." One could argue, which I do, that such philosophies are fundamental to the game and especially to the game of life. One could then question, which I also do, whether coaches really value their mentoring role or if their actions, rather than the governing infrastructure of the game itself—rules, umpires and referees, competition and results—provide the lasting off-field benefits of sports.

A common problem with early stage surveys is redundancy. They're constructed with excellent intentions, using rigorous design and post-analysis criteria, but they're inherently flawed by the simple fact that nobody ever gets anything right on the first try. Ironically, redundancy is also a strength of some surveys and can determine whether a respondent is answering truthfully or is at least consistent with their answers. Redundancy becomes a problem when the questions themselves are too similar or when they appear to address a similar topic, at least in the respondents' eyes. This often produces ambiguous results: everything looks the same and nothing or very little stands out.

Ambiguity was indeed a problem with the results as there was little variability in how each philosophy was ranked. For example, 9 of the 13 philosophies were ranked in the top 3 by 23 to 35% of coaches and teaching and mentoring philosophies overall were both ranked in the top 3 by 24%. What did stand out, however, were the four least popular philosophies: fair play, sportspersonship, learning from mistakes and winning.

I respect the coaches' delegation of winning to the bowels of youth sports philosophies, especially as a "build it (i.e., skills, team play, fitness, etc.) and they (i.e., wins) will come" approach is a proven model for success in athletics and almost every endeavor. I nevertheless find it disturbing that the three most important philosophies, in my opinion, those that are arguably the most likely to have lasting character-enriching consequences—fair play, sportspersonship and learning from mistakes—are the least valued by our youth coaches.

Although not a stated goal, the study also assessed coaching values from a different perspective by surveying training histories and interests. Comparing the two provides insight into their values because it demonstrates what they know, what they don't and what they want to improve, which we hope would address their inadequacies. For example, 86% of respondents have had some form of health and safety training while 56% would like additional training in topics such as CPR and basic first aid. A similarly high 80% have had training in the skills, tactics, communication and goals of the sport yet 70% want still more training in the "Xs and Os," 75% specifically in skills and tactics. This is contrasted by the 46% who have had no training whatsoever in "Coach beyond" topics like mental health, stress management, performance anxiety and mental toughness and by the 57% who want additional training.

The optimistic take on these results is that coaches are generally well trained in basic health and safety and in coaching the sport. It's also reassuring that well over half appear interested in improving their abilities regardless of topic. The pessimistic take is that most coaches primarily value the tangibles of coaching, the Xs and Os, over the intangibles that would substantially improve the on-field experience as well as the long-term benefits that stay with athletes for a lifetime. Realistically, these data aren't and shouldn't be surprising. Most youth coaches haven't participated in a formal certification program. Most of their knowledge arises from their own athletic experience and most coaches have limited if any understanding of teaching, not to mention mentoring, all of which was clearly substantiated by this study.

Were the respondents dishonest? Of course not. They're human, but honesty and truthfulness are not necessarily the same. I suspect respondents were honest with their intentions but possibly not consciously or even subconsciously truthful with their answers. Youth coaches are incredibly generous and for the most part motivated by love for the game, by personal connections to the kids, by community pride or by all of the above. They're clearly not incentivized financially with 41% working for free, according to the survey, and 75% working up to 23 hours a week for $0 to $5,000, not per week but for the entire season. Their interest in training is commendable and every sport's regulatory authority should do their best to accommodate such interests and by proxy the athletes' needs. Organizations should also pay for the training and certifications especially if they're not paying their coaches. Finally, the bill should feature prominently in such training, which could and should be guided by the survey results.

I coached youth baseball for a decade. I also coached youth track, mostly just my daughter, but also her high school indoor track team. My "formal" training consists of an online course by the Babe Ruth League, although I honestly don't remember if this included certification. I also participated in the Montgomery County Public School coach training program that consisted of one in-person coaching class and three health and safety classes, of which two were virtual. The general purpose of the courses was to identify and eliminate risks, to the athlete and to myself, and to manage difficult situations and health concerns. In my opinion, the baseball classes were structured to sincerely help the coach. The school classes, however, were structured to address liability concerns rather than teaching coaches how to coach. Yes, I'm a cynical person, but I also worked in academia for almost 29 years where I was required to take similar "liability relief" courses almost yearly; I know one when I see one.

Cynicism aside, all of the courses were helpful yet they were also grossly inadequate. I relied heavily on my professional experiences in academia and in my understanding of exercise physiology and biomechanics, luxuries that most youth coaches understandably lack. My approach was very different from that of my peers and my understanding of skills development was far superior, but my managing skills were weak in the beginning. In fact, neither I nor my peers had truly mastered the Holy Trinity, which I suspect is rare. Most were good at managing, some were good at teaching and almost none knew how to mentor.

Using a Holy Trinity grade scale where teaching, mentoring and managing are each assigned a perfect individual score of 1.0 and an average of 0.5, I'd rate my overall coaching acumen as a 2.3: 0.9 for teaching, 0.9 for mentoring and 0.5 for managing. I probably started at 1.7 (0.7 + 0.8 + 0.2) and through experience honed my teaching and mentoring skills and significantly improved at management. Most coaches learn to manage from experience, either from playing in college (hopefully), playing in high school (most likely) and/or from being a fan (hopefully not). Skills and scores should slowly improve with experience as mine did over a decade. They would improve far more rapidly, however, with training that I would estimate to give a 0.2 to 0.5 immediate bump to anyone's score.

My proposed Holy Trinity grading system is a subjective attempt to quantify coaching proficiency. Is it scientific? No, nothing subjective is scientific, but quantifying anything provides a means to evaluate and can convert subjectivity to objectivity when applied over time, assuming the grading scale remains constant. Do I propose its systemic use? Again no, although it would be flattering. I instead suggest employing a more constructive system that simply applies a numerical value to the Bill of Rights with, for example, 10 points/right and 5 for "average." School athletic directors, club managers and league administrators could then employ an objective system with internal controls for assessor variability, possibly with postscore rankings like the National Institutes of Health uses in evaluating grant applications. In this system, coaches' overall scores as well as those for each right would be ranked within each organizational unit, for example in a school or club, and the ranking rather than the scores would be used to compare coaches between units and even organizations. Rankings could also be used to identify coaching mentors and those with particular talents for advancing a specific right. The entire system could then be used to evaluate coaching staff, in advertising organizational excellence and, most importantly, to guarantee that coaches coach for the athletes' benefit rather than their own.

If you're wondering how my coaching colleagues and former athletes would think of my self-evaluated Holy Trinity ranking, well, so am I. No doubt some would object to a 2.3, arguing that I'm either suffering from delusions of grandeur or self-deprecation, but I'm pretty confident most would agree with my assessment. Coach evaluations were never performed and to be honest, I'm not sure such things even exist. A voluntary evaluation of my academic teaching can be read at the link provided here (https://www.ratemyprofessors.com/professor/1135267), although it represents only a tiny fraction of the students I taught over 14 years at Washington State and it doesn't include those at Johns Hopkins or Cal. It also has little direct relevance to coaching outside of generally demonstrating that I'm a pretty good teacher.

You're also probably wondering how I'd rate my colleagues and my children's current and former coaches. As expected, the collective group would receive about a 1.5, which is average. The range would span from 0.5 to 2.9, with Mike Hinz and Bob Freeman holding up the high end and a poorly trained and abusive father coach on the low end. I've coached with former Division I athletes and high school benchwarmers, with doctors and plumbers, with right-wing gun-toting zealots and tree-hugging tie-dye-wearing hippies and literally every one of them, including the abusive father, was committed to the kids and to the sport, or so they believed. Their actions may have betrayed their beliefs, but their intentions were universally admirable.

My children's school and club coaches would probably rank a little higher, but not by much. Some spent more time texting friends than running drills while others were annoyingly overcommitted, setting diets, checking bedtimes, offering dating advice and generally erasing boundaries, albeit with genuinely good intentions. Some coached club and high school teams, creating an obvious conflict of interest at the expense of their non-high school players. Others introduced Division I college-level training to a sixth-grade girls soccer team, practicing year-round in all weather conditions, employing drills, tactics and motivational strategies that I eventually realized were appropriate only for adults. Success was measured in championships and there were many as well as national rankings. Failure, by contrast, was evident in a collective psychosis that tore the team apart.

You're probably wondering which if any of these experiences typifies American youth sports. There's really no way of knowing, at least not without expanding programs like Project Play, although I'd be flabbergasted to learn that any were atypical as all of my negative experiences

Chapter 6

share a common malignancy: coaches coaching for themselves rather than the athletes. Notwithstanding, I do have contrasting examples that illustrate the challenges, successes and failures of two often encountered and diametrically opposed coaching approaches: the two Bryans.

Big Bryan played first base on a junior or community college baseball team. His playing career ended at this level and he began coaching when his son first started playing organized baseball, I believe when he was 8 years old, "playing up" in the Cal Ripken league. I never saw Big Bryan play, but his understanding of baseball was major league even if his playing skills weren't and his teaching skills were highly admirable, especially as he never had any formal training. He probably could have had an illustrious career as a college coach had he completed a bachelor's degree, but I doubt this ever entered his mind. He had a successful blue-collar job, a loving wife and he excelled at his passion of coaching youth baseball. He was content and I admired his commitment to the boys and the game.

Little Bryan wasn't little, just a lot smaller than Big Bryan and a lot more hairy. He played baseball in high school, which is where his playing career ended, and he started coaching in the Cal Ripken league as well. His understanding of baseball was typical of someone with little talent who hadn't played for a couple decades. He was a fine and respected coach in the community but lacked the baseball IQ to manage anything other than a local league team. He too had a successful blue-collar job, a loving wife, who by the way scared the bejesus out of me (love you Donna), and he was a natural leader of developing young men. He too was content and I admired his patience and respect for the boys.

Big Bryan had one son, pound for pound the best baseball player in town, regardless of age. He had an athletic build as a child and grew to be a strapping young man. He wasn't academically gifted, but his grades were good enough for the average state school and his prowess on the field was likely good enough to compensate for the few holes in his transcript. He was quiet if not introverted and had only a few close friends. Big Bryan coached his son's travel team and for all but a couple seasons let others, including myself, coach his son during league play for Cal Ripken and Babe Ruth. Both leagues evaluated and drafted their players annually and every year, Big Bryan's son was the top-ranked player.

The two had an interesting vicarious relationship that was apparent to everyone, including Big Bryan and the boy's mother who openly joked about it.

Little Bryan had two sons. The older was strong and athletic, highly coachable and good at every sport he played. The younger was the exact opposite: small and frail, textbook passive aggressive, utterly unaccomplished in anything athletic, completely un-coachable and afraid of his shadow. Younger was, however, creative, funny, highly social, extremely likeable and had a large friend group despite his awkwardness. Little Bryan coached most of Younger's teams, including once with my assistance. Younger was always the bottom-ranked player and coaches competed to avoid drafting him, not only due to his lack of talent but also because of the distractions he caused. He was terrified of the ball and wouldn't follow instructions, which created countless safety concerns. Little Bryan never appeared upset at Younger's on-field failures though and instead worked tirelessly to build his confidence and skills. Younger was terrified of the ball even as a teenager and would start inching out of the batter's box well before the pitch was thrown. "Stay in there 'Bud,' you can do it," Little Bryan would say and that front foot would hold steady. Their bond of trust was covalent.

So ask yourself, which Bryan would you want for a coach? Remember, the coach and son come as a complete package. With Big Bryan, you get the best player in town, the best coach in town and a guaranteed shot at the championship. With Little Bryan, you get a hole in the lineup, a walking error on the field and all too frequent emotional catastrophes. Championships aren't in the conversation, but fun is guaranteed. With Big Bryan, you get intensity, advanced drills and extra practices in a highly competitive atmosphere. Yes, he yells, but he also praises accomplishment, yielding a carrot and stick approach. With Little Bryan, you get patience and a comfortable learning environment that is de-stressed as much as possible. He never yells, always smiles and critiques rather than criticizes.

Be honest. If you're reading this book, you're likely a sports enthusiast and probably have a child currently playing at a competitive level, possibly even at an elite level or at a minimum considering a move to a

Chapter 6

travel team. Big Bryan is your choice. He was mine as well, in fact I chose coaches with similar approaches for both of my kids at all stages of their development . . . and it was a mistake. A regrettable, sometimes painful and, in hindsight, naïvely selfish mistake.

What motivated the Bryans and why were they coaching? Were they coaching for the athletes or themselves? This, I insist, is the most important consideration.

Coaches who coach for the athletes, who display empathy and are critical of themselves more than they are of their players/pupils, who are uncompromising in their commitment to developing their players rather than their own reputation, will always be successful. Success won't be measured with wins per se but by developing players to their fullest potential. Little Bryan lacked the technical skillset to coach at an advanced level and could have benefited greatly from formal training in tactics, strategy and skills. Nevertheless, he provided a safe and supportive learning environment that was loved by the boys and he incorporated others' advice, constantly looking to improve. He also exemplified the fundamentals of team coaching and leadership: never compromise another instructor's authority, always discuss conflicts away from pupils, delegate responsibilities and lead by example.

Big Bryan was the polar opposite of Little Bryan. He coached a relatively good travel team, but he never should have. He was prone to explosive outbursts and modeled poor to reprehensible behavior, clearly not understanding how to lead by example. Players, not umpires, were prime targets for his wrath as one had the power to penalize while the other was powerless. Typical bully behavior. Players and parents alike both feared and respected him, a common theme I've experienced among families hypnotized by the allure of winning coaches. His son not surprisingly bullied kids at school and was prone to emotional meltdowns in games. One happened after striking out to end an inning. He stood at the end of the dugout, quietly crying and trembling almost violently, as if in a seizure. The other boys ignored him, but my son was new to the team and tried consoling, "It's all right, man. It doesn't matter."

"Yes it does Freddie," the boy screamed, "It matters, it FUCKING MATTERS!"

Sympathy, pity and shame. The entire crowd felt all three, not only for the boy but for ourselves. We deserved it because nobody—not me, not the other coach, not the umpire, not even the boy's mother—intervened in any way. My son stood next to his friend for a moment and then headed to the field. Big Bryan's son quietly took off his helmet, grabbed his cap and glove and jogged to first base, never looking up from the ground. Big Bryan didn't say a word.

Big Bryan and I eventually had a heart to heart, not specifically about this incident but about coaching and his relationship with his son. He admitted his faults and took responsibility for what he defined as "harm." I believe he was sincere in his concern and in his guilt, although I don't think he recognized the systemic nature of his abuse, that it affected the entire team. He believed in altruism, that he sacrificed his time, money and energy to benefit his son, the team and the community it represented, but this was fallacy. He coached for himself, for the attention it provided among his peers, for the feeling of satisfaction and, from a Darwinian perspective, for his son's success. Every coach feels similar pressures and most succumb to them by differing degrees. Most, like Big Bryan, recognize and grow from their mistakes. It's important to understand that neither Bryan was paid for their services. This lack of compensation explains a false sense of altruism felt by many volunteer coaches, myself included. It also explains why paid coaches with professional training should be held to a higher standard, why their lapses can't be justified with false pretenses of altruism and why they are far less forgivable.

Coaching and mentoring draw many parallels to parenting. In fact, the basic philosophies and styles of parenting perfectly apply to both. First described by Diana Baumrind, who was an extremely accomplished professor of Psychology at the world's best academic institution, the University of California, Berkeley (Go Bears!), parenting styles fall into four basic categories: neglectful/uninvolved, indulgent/permissive, authoritarian and authoritative.[6] Dr. Baumrind originally proposed the latter three and adopted "neglectful" after considering the works of another stalwart in the field, Professor Eleanor Maccoby of Stanford University. The categories are oversimplifications, naturally, plastic examples used to better understand, study and treat behavior pathologies, yet they've stood the test of time since first proposed in the late 1960s and as theories are being revised to accommodate cultural differences, family dynamics and the bidirectionality of parenting (i.e., children's influences on parents).[7]

Authoritarian parents control everything. Rules are absolute and strictly enforced, children have no control or voice in decision making and negative reinforcement is primarily used to mold behaviors. Rules exist only on paper for indulgent parents who praise everything, criticize nothing and acquiesce with violations. Their children have never heard the word "no." The authoritative style falls in between with rules objectively enforced according to context. Children are encouraged and critiqued, again objectively, and openly participate in making decisions; they're valued contributors that recognize and respect their guiding authority. Neglectful parents let the inmates run the asylum.

Several coaching examples come to mind for each parenting style. The legendary Paul "Bear" Bryant, who won six national championships as head coach of the Alabama Crimson Tide football team, and Bobby Knight, who coached basketball at Army, Indiana, and Texas Tech and won over 900 games and three national championships, were also legendary authoritarians. Barry Switzer, another super successful head football coach with three national championships coaching the Oklahoma Sooners and a Super Bowl victory with the Dallas Cowboys, infamously gave his college players incredible freedom and epitomized the indulgent style during his professional coaching days. All of these coaches were successful, but at what cost?

Bryant didn't integrate his team until 1971, kicked players off for violating substance abuse rules he himself violated and infamously encouraged brutality in his practices and games. Bobby Knight and other coaches of that era often embraced a style that can only be described as abusive, both mentally and sometimes physically. Knight's anger mismanagement ultimately cost him his career as did that of Woody Hayes, Ohio State's very successful football coach from 1951 to 1978. I distinctly remember watching Hayes punch an opposing player in the neck just because the kid had the audacity to intercept OSU's quarterback. Switzer's college players were repeatedly in legal trouble for misdemeanor and felony charges including public intoxication, assault, drug trafficking, firing guns in the dorm and sexual assault. One of his most famous players, Brian "The Boz" Bosworth, described the program in his autobiography as bordering on anarchy. Switzer even admitted to covering up crimes through corrupt local officials and was forced to resign in 1989 due to his program receiving a three-year probation and 20 NCAA violations.

Authoritarian and indulgent coaching styles clearly produce mixed results with successes on the field and failures off. With parenting, the outcomes are remarkably similar to the off-field failures and are very well documented. Children raised in authoritarian households are more likely to be aggressive, display delinquent behaviors like substance abuse and crime as well as to develop anxieties. Similar delinquencies and aggression are associated with indulgent parenting and in addition, with anti-social behavior and impulse control. Basically, indulgent parenting produces brats. Neglectful parenting is generally described as the worst parenting style because it's associated with a high frequency of these and other negative outcomes as well as mental health/personality disorders including low self-esteem, anti-social behaviors, delinquencies, depression and anxieties. It's not surprising, therefore, that the analogous coaching styles can produce similar dysfunctions in players or even whole teams.

In contrast to each of these styles of parenting and coaching is the authori*tative* style, which was championed most notably by Jerry Tarkanian in an era dominated by authori*tarians*. It's a small difference in spelling but a major difference in practice. "Tark the Shark" racked up over 900 wins, a national collegiate championship and was elected to the Basketball Hall of Fame after coaching at so-called nobody schools. This includes three high schools, two community colleges and three universities that to be honest are only known to the sports world for employing Jerry: Long Beach State, Fresno State and the University of Nevada Las Vegas. He was renowned for creating success out of thin air, often where nobody noticed and with nobody players: kids from underrepresented and socially depressed communities, kids ignored by Division I programs, kids with little chance of success without strong mentoring, which Jerry provided. Honestly, how many of ESPN's Top-10 list of his players do you recognize?

1. Larry Johnson, UNLV
2. Stacey Augmon, UNLV
3. Armen Gilliam, UNLV
4. Sidney Green, UNLV
5. Reggie Theus, UNLV
6. Ed Ratliff, Long Beach State
7. Greg Anthony, UNLV
8. Eddie Owens, UNLV
9. J. R. Rider, UNLV
10. Freddie Banks, UNLV

Unlike the other parenting and coaching styles, the authoritative approach is associated with positive developmental outcomes like maturity, competence, high self-esteem and achievement. I seriously doubt Jerry was aware of this specific parenting style or if he knew anything about child developmental psychology. It appears, however, that his embrace of mentoring approaches that mirror authoritative parenting was a recipe for success, yet I'm saddened by the continued misunderstanding of coaching in today's youth sports, when I hear so much screaming or impenitent praise, when I read about the physical and mental abuses that have occurred in the Women's National Soccer League and when I witnessed firsthand similar abuses by Bear Bryant poseurs on my daughter's soccer team. It's time to end authoritarian and indulgent coaching.

Chapter 7

Toto, I've a Feeling We're Not in Idaho Anymore

The greatest movie of all time, regardless of genre, country of origin or cinematic movement, is undoubtedly *The Wizard of Oz*. The disagreeables among you need not share your obviously uninformed and sophomoric opinions because the rest of the physical and metaphysical universe has already voted.

The original book *The Wonderful Wizard of Oz* was written by Lyman Frank Baum and illustrated by William Wallace Winslow. It was the first in a series of 14 books exploring the mythical and mystical parallel universe of Oz that apparently can only be accessed via tornado, clipper ships to Australia and underground tunnels opened by earthquakes. Read the series and you'll understand.

Everyone knows the original story and everyone has seen the movie and although most have never read the series nor the founding book, it will probably surprise no one to learn that the movie wasn't entirely faithful to the book. As far as Hollywood transformations go, however, this one's actually pretty good, but some of the most famous lines in the movie never appeared in the book. This includes "Toto, I've a feeling we're not in Kansas anymore," which ironically is not only the most iconic line from the movie but also the most misquoted. "Toto, I have a feeling . . . ," "Toto, I've got a feeling . . . ," "Toto, I don't think we're . . ." You get the picture and I'm sure you know exactly what it means whenever you hear it.

Chapter 7

Moving from rural Idaho to a Washington, DC, suburb along the I-270 corridor was in many ways an Oz'ian experience for my children. My son was born in Los Angeles, but we moved to Pullman, Washington, shortly after his first birthday and then to Moscow, Idaho, when Meilani was born. They weren't exactly strangers to urban life and were in fact world travelers as we regularly visited friends in Seattle and in the San Francisco Bay area as well as relatives in Hong Kong, Dar es Salaam and the island of Zanzibar, but these were vacations. Both kids were nervous in crowds and surprisingly attentive to the differences walking among us. Homeless people disturbed and bewildered them, especially my son, and both kids were particularly sensitive to rudeness. People held open doors in Moscow and said "please" and "thank you." They raked their elderly neighbors' leaves in the fall and shoveled their driveways in winter. Doors were rarely locked, in houses or cars, and neighbors actually talked to each other, not with superficial pleasantries but with laughs and tears, over beers and barbecue, at the farmer's market and of course at ball games. Such intimacy is lost in cities even among our segregated tribes.

Things were different in Rockville. Better in most ways and not so much in others, although overall I believe the family would agree it was a good move. Moscow is a college town home to the University of Idaho and just seven miles from Washington State University in Pullman. The community is quaint and quiet with a small town American esthetic snuggled among the rolling hills of the Palouse, a multi-state region of grasslands in the Pacific Northwest. It's very small, very tight and very white. People of color were as rare as trees in the area, sprinkled across the campuses as faculty or students, mostly college athletes, as both universities struggled to increase diversity. Academics and townsfolk rarely mixed in the community even at times or places that would normally bring people together, like July 4 celebrations or the aforementioned farmer's markets or ball games, and although it's tempting to excuse the self-segregation to the off-putting hubris of overeducated faculty with a liberal arts defensiveness, this just wasn't the case. Academics are overzealous nerds not egocentric elitists. They're anxious to talk about their fields and research, they welcome difference, embrace diversity and absolutely adore disagreement, but any offense to their enthusiasm is misguided and usually self-imposed.

I was a professor for many years and I know these people well. I was also raised in a blue-collar household and lived in small farming towns until my college years, yet even I struggled for acceptance in Moscow. I had bona fides, mind you, rural credentials bolstered by having worked in the field rogueing and detasseling corn and bailing hay. I'm also an avid fisherman, fluent in the native tongue and was invited to participate in the most hallowed ceremonial duties of the tribe, coaching baseball, that is until the natives met my Chinese wife and *hapa* or *wasian* kids. I coached many years in Moscow and nobody was ever overtly rude, but introductions to my wife were always met with surprise and she never felt comfortable at games. Almost everyone was polite, but it doesn't take a genius to realize why invitations or greetings weren't reciprocated, why the players' parents never invited my wife to sit with them or why playdates were suddenly canceled after meeting her. In third grade, Meilani lost her best friend after the mother, who had been very friendly if not flirtatious with me, met my wife and if a reader suspects we're being oversensitive, the little girl admitted the mother didn't like Chinese.

My kids learned to recognize and deal with the subtle and not-so-subtle racism despite their young age. My son has always been a big dude, not especially tall, but barrel chested and very strong. If you're a fan of baseball, envision an Asian Kyle Schwarber with thick shaggy hair and eyebrows. He once responded to a kid making the "Asian face," pulling his eyelids shut, biting his lower lip with protruding incisors and saying, "Look, I'm Freddie Rodgers," by backhanding the boy's face with a Spider-Man lunchbox. No blood, no foul, just a confused and embarrassed young boy who learned a valuable lesson his parents should have taught.

Everything changed when we moved and my kids immediately felt at home in their new environment. Rockville, Maryland, is rich in diversity and is known as the capital's new Chinatown with many mixed-race households and with neighbors, restaurants and grocery stores to match my children's ancestry. Both played soccer and were eager to find new teams and friends, as were my wife and I, recognizing the experience would help with their transition into new schools that were five times larger than those in Moscow—another benefit of youth sports. Their teams were as diverse as the community with all manner of race and nationality represented. Why does this matter? Because they felt free to be themselves, to play and study with confidence, to not worry whether they were being judged from stereotypes rather than their performance on the field and in the classroom or by their character and, in addition, because my wife threw out Freddie's Spider-Man lunchbox when she opened it and found a garter snake.

I can understand why some conservatives believe that diversity has exaggerated or little value outside of increasing dining options. After all, I'm white and there was a time when I held the same belief. That was before I moved from Texas to Hawai'i, before I became a "minority," before I walked in their slippahs and let's face it, before I opened my mind and considered that maybe, just maybe my limited understanding of the world and its diversity of people, cultures and interests might not be the only one worthy of consideration and respect. I learned that *Locals* and *Local Motion* are brand names in Hawai'i, but "locals only" is an ideology, one that isn't unique to an island population of mostly Asian and mixed Asian people but also to the predominantly (entirely?) white ski towns in Northern Idaho. Both communities garnish pickup trucks, tee shirts and baseball caps with the words "locals only" and both seek to distinguish themselves from the invading tourist hordes in a defiant expression of cultural identity, but neither are expressing racism. They are, however, expressing tribalistic protectionism, whether justified or not, as well as the safety one feels in a like-minded group.

My children's most significant Oz'ian experiences, however, were unrelated to racial diversity and, as I think you'll eventually agree, were probably inversely related to it. Talent and the level of competition in the DC metro area (aka DMV for DC/Maryland/Virginia) were the biggest surprise and far exceeded our expectations. Before the move, both kids played in travel and local leagues for different sports, both had experience playing against teams from much larger communities like Spokane, Washington, and Boise, Idaho, and both fully expected to encounter more, better and more better athletes when we moved. Our surprise came not from the disparity in talent, which we all suspected, but from the magnitude of difference and from the underlying cause: money.

The fact is that many urban youth sports communities are dominated by leagues of privilege: expensive travel teams composed of players from wealthy to very wealthy families with seemingly endless resources like private practice facilities, professional coaches, personal trainers, the most expensive equipment and gear and the economic freedom to travel anywhere, including overseas. Socioeconomic disparity, not racial diversity, was the greatest and most surprising difference between our former and new home. It defined our experiences in many ways and, as we learned, is symptomatic of a national trend.

Moscow and Pullman each had recreational leagues for different sports that were managed by their local governments as well as separate youth baseball and football associations. Private non-profit travel soccer clubs were also available, one for each community, and the region shared a highly successful youth track club, the Pullman Comets. Ice hockey, lacrosse, gymnastics and travel teams for other sports also existed, but participation was too small to support local leagues so travel was a necessity. Participation was also too small to support more than one travel team for each age group so some were consolidated. In fact, younger teams were often composed of both boys and girls of different ages and although most teams were segregated by sex, boys' and girls' teams often played one another. This made for grand entertainment especially when a girls' team dominated.

Rockville is typical of most relatively wealthy urban communities with access to a plethora of organized clubs and for a variety of sports. Each is staffed with professional coaches and some own or lease specialized facilities. The more elite clubs or those with established histories also require certification for most of their coaches who rapidly acquire experience from coaching multiple teams, of multiple age groups at multiple skill levels. It's difficult to appreciate the difference in scale between Moscow and Rockville or between any urban and rural community without relevant examples so consider soccer, not all sports, but just soccer.

The Maryland State Youth Soccer Association lists 195 separate soccer clubs in the state: 81 within a 20-mile radius encompassing

Chapter 7

Rockville and 12 within 5 miles. This is compared to just 2 clubs on the Palouse, an area over 18,000 square miles. I'm likely missing a couple clubs, especially as the Pullman and Moscow clubs aren't even listed with their states' youth soccer websites, but this alone is telling. The largest club serving the Rockville area is Montgomery Soccer Inc. or MSI Soccer, named after Montgomery County. It manages leagues for beginner, recreational and developing or "classic" athletes in addition to travel/academy teams. It also manages a league for special needs athletes and holds multiple tournaments and showcase events for multiple age groups and stratified skill levels that attract teams from throughout the Mid-Atlantic. MSI alone registers over 10,000 athletes. For a little perspective, this is equivalent to the entire student body of the University of Idaho or the permanent population of Pullman, which according to the recent census has a population of 33,508 of which approximately 28,000 are university students and temporary residents, most of whom disappear in the summer and don't have kids playing soccer.

Finding teams for my children or even trying to understand the nomenclature and structure of the different leagues and organizations around Rockville was dizzying. I literally spent hours scouring websites, scrutinizing clubs, quizzing administrators and emailing coaches and league directors. Tryout locations were scattered throughout the county on school fields, in city parks and at one of youth soccer's nicest facilities, the Maryland SoccerPlex with 21 outdoor immaculately manicured grass fields (aka pitches) that looked more like 100-meter putting greens, three modern artificial turf pitches with stadium lighting, an indoor fieldhouse with two turf fields and Maureen Hendrick's Field at Championship Stadium, former home to the Washington Spirit and Champion of the National Women's Soccer League. In Moscow, I filled out a form, mailed a check and walked my kids down to the middle school.

Teams in Montgomery County had already filled by the time we moved and summer seasons were well underway yet I was still contacted by probably a dozen coaches with tryout offers. Were they thirsty for talent or fees? I'm sure they wanted both, but I wasn't in a position to care and although the price tag was shocking—four times what we paid in Moscow, creating my own Oz'ian experience—our two professional salary household could afford it. Many families in the area can't, however, and although the larger clubs offer scholarships, I've never met or known a beneficiary. In fact, competitive rankings within any of these organizations appear to scale perfectly with average household incomes, at least based on the cars waiting for practices to end, the zip codes of the families and the number of children enrolled in highly expensive private schools. The system is structured according to class where children from lower-income families play on recreational teams, middle class play classic and wealthy play at the "competitive" level, on travel and academy teams. There are of course exceptions as well as families that irresponsibly bet the farm, so to speak, hoping that an investment now will attract scholarships and professional offers later in life. Parents and coaches discussed the issue openly and it's been well documented by journalists, most notably by Linda Flanagan who wrote *Take Back the Game: How Money and Mania are Ruining Kids' Sports—and Why It Matters*, which in my opinion is an excellent and required read for anyone contemplating competitive club sports for their children.

Flanagan is personally connected to the topic through running and coaching and professionally through associations with the Aspen Institute, the Positive Coaching Alliance and her many writings. This book and other writings discuss the competitive sports toll on child athletes, from overtraining injuries, bullying and psychological burnout to the financial and emotional costs on what Flanagan describes as the enabling "unpaid support network," the families. Her works chronicle what she and others consider problems in the field, but because they focus on the problems, sometimes exclusively, readers can be easily misled into tossing the baby out with the bathwater. Anecdotal evidence is used far too often, symptomatic of journalism rather than science, and some of her referenced academic studies are highly preliminary or too specific for generalizing. This is her schtick, her specialization, and she's adept at selling her message, but even she admits that playing is far better than not and she rightly highlights some disturbing trends that all parents and athletes should consider.

She and others cite a 2019 market analysis of youth sports conducted by WinterGreen Research that estimated its global size to be

$24.9 billion, the United States contributing $19.2 billion. The projected global market was expected to exceed $76 billion by 2026 or $60 billion in the United States if market growth rates similarly tracked. The Aspen Institute suggests that the rates do indeed track as their independent analysis in 2022 placed the US market between $30 and $40 billion. These numbers probably underestimate the total youth sports market that not only includes team membership and fees, software subscriptions, travel expenses, equipment, facility rentals and capital improvements, all of which were addressed, but also apparel and footwear, consultants and private coaching as well as overlap with related markets like nutritional supplements. Perspective check number 2: the National Football League market was only valued at $15 billion in 2019.

It may or may not surprise you to learn that youth sports is big business and even if you've read the writings of Flanagan or others in the field or if you're a professional coach, you're probably unaware of just how big it is or even how successful your local non-profit club can be. Only one of our regional clubs publishes an annual financial report, the Arlington Soccer Association of Arlington, Virginia, and although I requested reports from other clubs in our area, only Arlington cooperated. Good on you Arlington!

This is another large non-profit club with 501(c)(3) tax status and approximately 9,000 registered athletes playing on 640 teams. Their top travel teams play in the Elite Clubs National League or "ECNL," which is arguably the best and most selective league in the country. Arlington also manages travel teams in other less competitive but still respectable leagues. In fact, 45% of their athletes play on travel or elite teams. Such diversification is typical of large clubs, although how each club prioritizes resources and development of recreational, travel and elite teams often varies as, for example, with MSI that prioritizes low/beginning- and high/classic-level recreation over travel.

In 2022, Arlington generated $7,555,500 in revenue. Their expenses were primarily limited to salaries and staff, which ate 73% of their budget. Operations gobbled 23% and financial aid the remaining 4% for a total of $6,127,500 and a net profit of $1,428,000. That's a net profit margin of 18.9%. When this is compared to the net margin rankings for different business sectors, a list compiled by New York University Professor of Finance Dr. Aswath Damodaran, and if we assume Arlington's profit margins are typical of club soccer, we arrive at perspective check number 3: the sector ranks 15th in the country sandwiched between coal and related energy and the pharmaceutical industry as well as 77 positions above consumer and office electronics.

If you're wondering how a small local non-profit can generate over $1.4 million with a net profit rate equivalent to Eli Lilly's yet only provide $250,500 or 17% of their profits in financial aid, you're not alone. Many have criticized sports clubs as well as the entire youth sports industry for establishing a pay-to-play class system that largely ignores families in lower socioeconomic brackets, including Linda Flanagan who rightly points out that youth soccer is the worst of the worst. In two articles published in *The Atlantic*, "The Downsides of America's Hyper-Competitive Youth-Soccer Industry" (July 13, 2018) and "What's Lost When Only Rich Kids Play Sports" (September 28, 2017), Flanagan describes a sport and industry designed to maximize profits at the expense of families where finances, priorities, vacations, education and even relationships are affected. She describes a system structured not for the development of elite athletes per se but wealthy elite athletes raised mostly by educated parents with professional salaries and a surplus of time and money, where families fly 10-year-old children cross-country to play in "elite" tournaments, often in name only, and spend thousands if not tens of thousands of dollars every year on their child's hobby. Even the costs of college recruiting now fall on parents.

Whereas scouts and coaches from other sports still attend high school games and club tournaments, soccer scouting primarily occurs at team showcases and identification or "ID" camps held by the college coaching staff or by leagues and clubs, all for a hefty fee. Many if not most of these events are overtly commercial with very little scouting. League and club events are often attended by very few and sometimes no outside coaches or by coaches from obscure programs seeking even a modicum of recognition. College camps can be worse, dream sinks with only guest appearances from head coaches who pay little to no attention to the athletes. I've attended more than a few, for baseball and soccer, and while some coaches readily admit interest in only a few preselected athletes, most are true to the charade.

The Aspen Institute's Parenting Survey documented this class disparity and was authored by two academics, Dr. Travis Dorsch of Utah State University and Dr. Jordan Blazo of Louisiana Tech University, neither of whom have a dog in the fight. The study was financed by TeamSnap, a software company that develops applications for managing teams and leagues and that has an invested interest in understanding parents' needs and desires. As you might have guessed, children from the richest households were twice as likely to play on club travel teams with 44% from households making over $150,000 and 20% making below $50,000. Soccer players represented the largest fraction in the Parenting Survey at 26.5% or 523 families. When respondents were partitioned by household income, the wealth stratification of soccer families was the third worst among the different sports and was skewed disproportionately toward the upper end with 35% in the $100,000+ bracket, twice the percentage for any other earning bracket. Only lacrosse and swimming were more skewed, although they together represented only 2.7% of respondents.[1] Soccer, traditionally an international sport for the poor and bourgeoisie, has become a pastime for American aristocrats whose preferred playground is the ECNL.

The ECNL is truly a national league, one of three with boys' and girls' teams from all but 15-ish states depending on the year. It was founded in 2009 as a girls' league with the intent of emulating the training environments and rigor of European youth leagues. It rapidly expanded and drew talent away from smaller regional leagues partly due to an organization structure where clubs rather than teams join the league. Boys' clubs were added in 2017 while both boys' and girls' teams further expanded when the US Soccer Development Academy of the United States Soccer Federation folded. This seminal event also gave rise to the other national leagues: MLS Next, a boys-only league linked to Major League Soccer and the Girls Academy. Both attract elite talent, both are highly competitive and both provide development services to help athletes land coveted college scholarships. However, both are also chasing the ECNL in many regards.

The ECNL is subdivided into national and regional leagues with usually one team from each club in each league. National league teams are the better of the two and travel across the country for championship tournaments, assuming they qualify, and because there's money to be had almost everyone qualifies. Regional league teams are still very competitive, but travel for league play is limited to a particular region, which doesn't include non-league tournaments. As of 2023, the ECNL club directory lists 128 and 144 girls' national and region teams, respectively, and 144 and 148 boys' teams. Teams are organized by age groups and each club has six national and regional teams.

Annual player registration fees for joining an ECNL team can vary greatly and have been rumored to reach the $10,000 range. Those in the DMV charged about $3,000 when Mei played, which, based on a quick internet search, is pretty typical but not all inclusive. Uniforms, tournament costs, special equipment and other fees are almost always added throughout the season. Clubs are tight lipped about fees and generally won't reveal even the registration fees until an offer is made. At which time, the player is pressured to immediately accept the offer that subsequently expires in one or two days. This practice is common for most travel teams, not just ECNL teams, and is in my personal opinion despicable. It makes it utterly impossible to critique the coaching, to assess the team personality, to learn about club dynamics and, most importantly, to predict your child's fit within the overall program.

In order to estimate the ECNL financial market, I began by surveying 48 randomly chosen teams to estimate the number of players per team for each age group. The younger teams registered on average 16 players while the middle and high school teams averaged 24. I then multiplied the assumed $3,000 registration fee to the approximate number of players for the entire ECNL system to estimate the total revenue generated by ECNL registration fees at $231,072,000. Keep in mind that this estimate represents only the tip of the total ECNL club market as it doesn't include tournament, showcase or ID camp costs or many other related fees and expenditures. Adding another $1,000 per person to accommodate some of these additional expenditures, which I can personally assure you is a conservative figure, brings the total estimate to $249,280,000.

Chapter 7

Don't confuse this astounding figure with ECNL valuation, a measure of corporate net worth. The organization's value is considerably lower with a reported league revenue of $3.4 million in 2019, according to the 2022 *Washington Post* article "Where Girls Compete but Men Rule" by Molly Hensley-Clancy. Because ECNL registration fees are parsed between clubs and leagues where they cover legitimate overhead costs, my estimates instead reflect the total amount of money involved in registering players and teams within the ECNL system. Factoring in travel expenditures, uniforms, practice gear, medical bills and private coaches to approximate the total out-of-pocket expenditures for ECNL families would likely approach if not eclipse $1 billion. In fact, the "triple it" rule of thumb is commonly quoted by parents when asked how registration fees compare to the total cost of playing on an elite travel team. Perspective check number 4: this is just one national league for just one sport that isn't even the most popular in the country.

We were unprepared for the commerciality of "big soccer" when we moved to Rockville. I expected it to be expensive and I expected and enthusiastically welcomed the structured bureaucracy of the different clubs, but the wealth and prosperity of the DMV soccer market did and continues to astonish me. My wife was raised in Hong Kong and educated in London. She's dumbfounded by the American fascination with sports and rolls her eyes with every written check. She also frequently, rightly and thankfully vetoes some of my and my children's spending desires, but for the most part allows me to manage our children's athletic careers. Her influence is grounding and welcomed but unfortunately all too uncommon in most American households and especially in lower-income households. The Parenting Survey suggests that those making less than $50,000 annually paid on average $544 for their child's sports over the previous year. This may only be 1% of the upper income for this bracket, but some of these families paid over $17,000, which is minimally 35% of the household income.

It's tempting to criticize these families as most journalists writing in this space have done. Such criticism, however, is low-hanging fruit. I think most people would agree that investing 35% of any household income, no matter its size, toward athletic training for your child is extremely irresponsible, from a personal finance perspective and from a general parenting perspective, unless modeling privilege and narcissism is your goal. Most people would also question the motivation of any such investment and wouldn't be surprised to learn that these families cite college athletic scholarships as the principal reason for their investment. Could this be justified by 35% of the household income on sports? Probably not, but what about a modest investment, say the average for this bracket? At what level is an investment into your child's athletic development advantageous or detrimental to their overall development?

The most common educational investment is the 529 college saving plan. These tax-free plans are offered by every state and Washington, DC, and their performance can be estimated from historical trends using online calculators that are widely available. Using the calculator on the US Office of Financial Readiness revealed that investing $544 annually with a 7% rate of return and an assumed 4.8% education cost inflation rate, which are standard assumptions for these calculators, would generate only $6,683 over a child's typical eight-year playing time. This covers just 2.6% of the estimated $253,678 needed to afford an average four-year in-state college. My cost assumptions included a starting tuition of $22,839 provided by the College Board's *Trends in College Pricing 2022*, and a room and board estimate of $17,730 provided by the Office. Investing $5,000 a year would cover only 24%, which makes the average $3,000 investment in DMV teams look pretty darn good, at least that's what I tell my wife. All of this naturally assumes your child is among the high school athletes who are athletically and academically accomplished enough to obtain a scholarship. So what's the magic percentage? According to the NCAA, only 2%.

We met one of these 2%'ers on Mei's first day of practice in the DMV. "Diana Prince" was only 9 years old, playing up on a team of elder yet mere mortals. How did I know she would eventually play collegiate soccer for an NCAA Division I program? I didn't, at least not for sure, but she literally stood a head above the other girls despite being younger. She also had Hermes' speed, Hercules' strength and the hyper-competitiveness of an amalgamated Michael Jordan and Tom Brady. She was the daughter of two former NCAA Division I athletes, a wide

Chapter 7

receiver for the Naval Academy and a sprinter for Howard University, and she had played on the national youth team for her age group and won multiple ECNL accolades. Her elder sister was a high school soccer star and played for the Naval Academy while her middle school brother was being scouted by top collegiate programs. Anyone not jealous of the family's superior genetics and universal accomplishments needs counseling and if the entire family wasn't so dang smart, nice and well adjusted, I'd hate them all.

Diana's mother introduced herself when we first arrived. The girls hadn't yet developed the adolescent insecurities that complicate introductions and immediately started passing and juggling the ball, occasionally emitting a whisper or giggle. The mother was gregarious and blunt, a lot like Mei, and a pleasant and insightful source of DMV soccer information. Her eldest child had already played in the system for many years and her clairvoyance would prove invaluable to Mei and me navigating the system.

Mei and Diana couldn't have been more different. Mei was tiny, Diana mighty. Mei was a dribbler and master of the game's technical skills while Diana was power incarnate. They never developed a deep friendship but were the dynamic duo on the pitch. In a typical game, Diana would score five or six goals and Mei would score two or three while assisting on half of Diana's. I never heard a complaint from other kids or parents as everyone appeared content with how games progressed. The team won every league game, every tournament and one of two league championships.

Mei and Diana had announced that they were leaving the classic team for more competitive travel clubs. The coach begged us to remain and offered to waive the fees if we "double carded," which allows kids to play on separate teams in different leagues. The announcement devastated team dynamics and in hindsight was a mistake, although I'm not sure it could have been avoided. All the families knew we were "exploring options" and we were constantly asked about our searches. Many wondered why we'd leave given the girls' privileged positions on the team. "Because that's what you do," Diana's mother said and to be honest, I simply followed her advice because if I wanted something better for

Mei, if she wanted something better for herself and she did, in fact she vehemently begged to play on a travel team, this really is what you do.

We soon learned that Diana would be joining the Maryland Rush Montgomery or "MRM" Coyotes, a travel team that played in the top bracket of the Elite Development Program or "EDP" regional league, eventually joining the US Youth Soccer National League. Rush claims to be the largest international soccer organization with 91 clubs in the United States and 65 globally, while the EDP is generally recognized as good, but not great, at least compared to the ECNL. The USYS National League, however, is excellent and provides competition equivalent to the top teams in the ECNL.

Mei first tried out for the MSI Academy team and later for the Coyotes. Compared to her former team, the Academy was noticeably more aggressive on and off the ball. They played physically, pushing, shoving and tackling the ball and were all around better athletes. One girl had advanced ball skills on par or even superior to Mei's, but nobody matched Mei's speed. The girls immediately accepted her, were warm and welcoming and the coach pulled her aside to extend an offer.

Mei was beaming. She demanded we accept the invitation and continuously argued its merits over the entire ride home. I too was thrilled. The Academy represented a big step forward in competition and hopefully in coaching, although I remained agnostic. The tryout itself was a bit disorganized and the coaching was limited to drills as the girls mostly scrimmaged. I also couldn't shake the feeling that I was being sold, not from the start but from the moment the coach started to pay attention to Mei. Was this good or bad? Should I expect a coach to be skeptical or enthusiastic? The invitation was a pleasant surprise, but would a quality program really extend an offer so quickly?

The Coyotes didn't hold organized tryouts. Instead, they invited players to attend a normal practice and because the team was the best in the Mid-Atlantic region, hopefuls often drifted in and out of practice and were for the most part ignored by the Coyotes. They were good and they knew it. They also knew very few could compete at their level and most girls never returned for a second practice.

Chapter 7

Coyotes' practices were highly structured, with formalized warm-up routines and skills-developing exercises. The latter built upon each other, first focusing on fundamental skills like juggling, dribbling, passing and receiving a pass, then intermediate skills like dribbling and passing when challenged and finally team skills like mini-scrimmages and full team scrimmages. One of two coaches, "Dr. Henry Jekyll," led the practice because he and the other coach, "Mr. Hyde," managed four teams for Rush: "A" and "B" teams for the 2005 and 2006 age groups. Jekyll was highly competent, critical yet fair in critique. We would eventually learn that he was also a classic enabler, refusing to address the team's pathologies, principle of which was Hyde. The latter was equally competent but incapable of critique and provided only monstrous criticism and often reprehensible behavior. They together possessed a bipolarity only Robert Louis Stevenson could describe.

Jekyll treated Mei as if she was already on the team. I'm not sure he complimented anything she did, but he would immediately correct mistakes regardless of who made them. This is a common and thoroughly successful teaching technique that prevents formation of bad habits and guides students, in this case athletes, to learn from their mistakes. It can be intimidating, especially when corrections are made publicly among a crowd of judgmental strangers, but it was expected at this level of play. In fact, I wholeheartedly welcomed it and recognized it for what it was, good coaching.

Mei excelled in the 1-versus-1 or "1-v-1" drills no matter who she faced. Jekyll noticed and gradually moved her from lower to higher skilled groups and she held her own. Scrimmaging was a different beast altogether as the speed and aggressiveness was like nothing she had ever experienced. She was kicked, scratched and grabbed as she struggled in challenges and although she managed well on the ball, she couldn't defend and didn't understand how to move off the ball. She was an excellent athlete who had never been properly coached. At one point, she took a pass over the middle, cutting, juking and carving her way to the goal when a girl from the older 2005 team, who was quite literally twice her size, blasted into her shoulder and launched her airborne. Mei hit the ground hard, landing on her back and sliding into a patchwork of grass, mud and gravel. Play briefly stopped, not to console Mei but the crying defender whose bloodied nose was elbowed during the collision and, to my surprise, resumed after only a few seconds and a quick word by Jekyll. The players were silent. They didn't flinch or blink or appear to care even superficially about the injured players. They instead resumed play while Mei jumped back on the proverbial horse.

She acted like nothing happened, but I knew it bothered her. Mei wasn't physically tough, at least not yet, and although she was born with a razor-sharp wit, cunning creativity and the defense mechanisms of a threatened momma grizzly bear, she was a baby when hurt. Jekyll complimented her toughness after practice and noted her successes on the ball, but she wasn't buying it. He was good, he knew how to teach and she admitted the Coyotes were a far better team, but she wanted nothing to do with them. The hit added to what she perceived was a personal attack. None of the girls talked to her during practice unless scolding her mistakes. They whispered and giggled conspicuously and one girl in particular fixated on her with a continuous and menacing glare. Mei never felt welcomed. It was business only from the precise moment she stepped onto the field.

Jekyll extended an offer after the practice and Mei was stunned. She didn't understand why everyone was so cold or why they "beat her up" during the scrimmage. She felt slighted and humiliated, which was entirely misplaced as she played very well, but she didn't see it that way. Nothing I said could have convinced her otherwise and she chose the Academy, a decision she and I would soon regret.

Remember that we left our classic team for better coaching and for the opportunity to experience elite competition. What we got, however, was a disinterested lazy coach glued to his phone and mediocre competition. More often than not, he'd show up late for games with parents and the team manager substituting in a panic. His practices were dull and uncreative and it was apparent to me that he was biding time. Parents frequently complained about his phone habits and organized an intervention that he countered with irreverence, telling Mei, the team's leading scorer, to stop shooting. It was a vindictive attempt to hurt the team, a proverbial punt on first down.

Chapter 7

Mei didn't take a shot over the next four games and the team lost all of them. This was the only time during her entire youth soccer career that she cried after a game and it broke my heart. I promised we could change teams if she finished the season unhappy. I then broke a cardinal rule of parenting youth athletes by inserting myself as coach, substituting for his supposed expertise and telling her to ignore everything he said and just shoot. The team again started winning and she finished the season with an astounding 36 goals.

True to Mei's competitive spirit, she was ready to jump ship at season's end. She loved her Academy teammates and I loved the parents. They were collectively the best sports family of both my children's teams and we still remain close to some of them. Nevertheless, the taste of mediocrity had spoiled Mei's appetite for fun. She wanted to be coached properly and to be properly challenged, so I gave Jekyll a call.

CHAPTER 8

Killing Coyotes

I saw my first coyote when I was a child. We were dove hunting and the animal trotted along the horizon moving to my left, stopping briefly to examine something on the ground before disappearing behind the brush. At the time, we lived in Mississippi or maybe Arkansas and I was a regular to the woods, grassy fields and muddy ponds where I usually hunted crows and snakes with a BB gun better suited for playing "BB tag" than killing animals. This time was an exception. I was carrying a 16-gauge shotgun, a beginner's weapon, but hadn't fired it all day, which is probably why I remember the coyote. Over the coming years, I saw several coyotes in Iowa, Texas, California and Maryland, but these were solitary and uneventful sightings. My first real introduction to a coyote pack and to its cunning, relentless, coordinated and unmercifully violent attacks occurred when we moved to the Palouse.

You hear them crying at night, like a small child. It's spooky and nothing like anything depicted in westerns. The first time we heard it, my wife was convinced a lost child was wailing somewhere in the neighborhood and stood searching through the window until one wailing child turned into two and then many. The next morning, we learned that a neighbor's golden retriever had been lured into the hills and killed by the pack. A couple years later, we awoke to a defiant screech, the sound of scratching nails along the cement and a couple short monomaniacal growls. I looked out the window and saw the blackened silhouette of two mid-size dogs playing tug-of-war with the neighbors' cat. By the time I got to the balcony, the coyotes were gone and peace had returned, at least until my neighbor discovered the blood-stained driveway and the remains of a single paw.

Coyotes by themselves are unimpressive in their predatory attributes. Like wolves, they'll feed primarily on small rodents when hunting alone but transform into legions of stormtroopers when hunting as a pack. They're incredibly agile, fast and intelligent and they attack with black-op coordinated precision, sophistication and ferocity unburdened by domestication. My 100+ pound Rhodesian ridgebacks are notorious hunters and I've seen them in fights with other large dogs including a Great Dane and once two Akitas at the same time, winning with ease and quite proud of their accomplishment. I have no doubt they could and would kill a single coyote with similar ease. I also have no doubt they'd experience the same fate as my neighbors' pets in an unbalanced encounter.

Every game the MRM Coyotes played was an unbalanced encounter. They were as agile, fast, intelligent and ferocious as a pack of real coyotes and had, by the time Mei joined them, already established themselves as a national powerhouse in both GotSoccer rankings and in winning prestigious tournaments. Rankings can be misleading of course with some teams building points through mass action, winning cupcake tournaments and playing in cupcake leagues, but the Coyotes played in the highest EDP regional league and won tournaments normally dominated by the best ECNL teams. They would accumulate tens of thousands of points over a season, often exceeding the state's runner-up by 5- or 10-fold.

The Coyotes were playing a friendly against a team from Northern Virginia and Jekyll had already seen Mei's technical skills but had only seen her scrimmage on a half-sized field so he invited her to try out in the friendly. It was not a particularly good day; it was cold, dark and raining, in the late winter and with barren treetops fading into the low-hanging black clouds. The streetlamps had turned on automatically despite it being mid-day and the parking lot was essentially a bog. We arrived early to find the entire Coyote team warming up in the rain with their parents waiting under trees and umbrellas. This was contrasted by our opponents, most of whom had not arrived while the few that had were huddled in the warmth of their parents' minivans and SUVs. This was also my introduction to the team's defining dynamic hyper-competitiveness among players and parents alike.

Two other girls were also trying out and they too arrived comparatively late, at least by Coyote standards. Both were bigger than all but one of the Coyotes, while Mei looked like someone's younger sister, easily the smallest on the field. The game itself was by any measure the fastest, most aggressive and most professional youth soccer game I had seen by then. For me, it was a mesmerizing introduction to elite club soccer and to its unmatched intensity, something my Academy friends still don't comprehend, while for Mei it was an immersion into chaos. Everyone was fast, everyone could dribble and everyone was physical. Mei was probably the fastest girl on the pitch and handled the ball well, but her misunderstanding of the game, of where and how to move when not possessing the ball, was glaringly apparent. Late in the game, however, she received a cross at the top of the box, took a small touch and blasted the ball between a diving goalie and the near post, helping the Coyotes to a 3–0 victory.

Jekyll liked what he saw. He was also surprisingly blunt in his criticism, not mean or rude as the gruffness of his game-time demeanor had disappeared, but unemotionally direct, both calculated and balanced in his praise and criticism. He concluded his objective assessment with an invitation to join the team, a golden ticket. Any doubt or concern I had regarding Mei's reception to her first professional critique were extinguished the moment I saw her smile.

Only one of the other girls also joined the team, "Arya Stark," a defensive player who normally played center back. She was aggressive and fast but like Mei didn't understand the game and according to Jekyll, both would require significant work. They were also told not to expect a starting role or to see much if any playing time in the near future. Mei accepted the contention as a challenge, resolute in becoming the team's starting striker, and spent hours juggling the ball, passing against the basement wall and practicing turns. She was balancing indoor track practices with her club track team, the Firebirds, while on off days practicing soccer with the Coyotes, either in middle school gymnasiums or on empty tennis courts in the freezing cold. Her devotion was commendable and Jekyll and Hyde had noticed, complimenting her growth and improved physical play. All was going swimmingly well until I opened my big mouth.

I told them we'd miss a couple practices for a track meet and was met with cold, silent stares. Hyde finally spoke, admitting that he didn't know she ran track. Jekyll said he thought that was over, permanently. Hyde asked what events she ran and why. Jekyll asked if we planned to keep running track. Neither were smiling.

I naïvely expected praise and adulation for their newfound gem and future striker, a devoted athlete who was mature beyond her years and was diligently and responsibly training in a complementary sport, one that would substantially improve her soccer abilities and potentially the Coyotes. I also assumed that as professional coaches, they were well aware that sports specialization increases risks for overuse injury, re-injury after rehabilitation and burnout in young athletes, whereas sports diversification has precisely the opposite effect while improving athletic performance. Other parents overheard the conversation and called me later to commiserate, explaining that they were similarly confronted over their daughters' conflicted interests. The team unofficially forbade playing multiple sports, which resulted in ultimatums and players quitting or being asked to leave. Total commitment was expected despite its detriment to the athlete.

This was the first of many conflicts that would come to symbolize the Coyotes experience: conflicts between the coaches, players and/or parents, conflicts with referees and tournament managers, conflicts over playing time and position, conflicts over real and perceived favoritism and, worst of all, conflicts over rampant bullying. Something was always amiss yet the problems and problematic people were never addressed. Jekyll and Hyde constantly modeled unprofessional and often malicious behavior, insulting and degrading players, verbally assaulting referees, physically assaulting equipment, throwing sideline tantrums and tirades. Worst of all, they managed by fear, not respect, nurturing an environment of distrust and bullying.

Most parents excused the abuse—and it was definitely abuse—as a "the price for greatness." Some accepted it as "character building" while denigrating other parents and players who had the audacity to complain. It created a toxic environment on and off the field where some parents, I'm convinced, encouraged if not urged malicious bullying. I became "that guy," confronting the coaches and calling out parents when societal taboos and mores were so clearly violated, yet I too drank the Kool-Aid, ultimately failing my daughter and exposing her to misogynistic insults as well as to subtle physical and not-so-subtle emotional attacks.

Our experience unfortunately appears to be more typical than not. In fact, misogyny and abuse in girls youth soccer infiltrates higher levels of play, as with women's professional soccer, and in more insidious ways. Molly Hensley-Clancy has written extensively on the topic as a sports investigative journalist for the *Washington Post* and formerly for *Buzzfeed*. This includes a recent article documenting FIFA's struggles to curtail sexual harassment and abuse of female soccer players in Haiti and Argentina, noting that serious allegations have also surfaced in Afghanistan and Zambia and that women and adolescent girls were victimized.[1] She and other reporters have most famously written about systemic abuses in the National Women's Soccer League or "NWSL" that included verbal and emotional abuse as well as "sexual misconduct" with allegations of assault, harassment and *quid pro quo* propositions for playing time.

These allegations first surfaced in an article published by *The Athletic*,[2] where journalist Meg Linehan described several disturbing encounters between Paul Riley, the league's winningest coach at the time, and two former players. The league failed these and countless unknown players by ignoring reports leading to Riley's departure from the Portland Thorns as well as others that eventually purged half of the league's head coaches by the season's end. The US Soccer Federation followed the season with an investigation led by Sally Yates, the former US attorney and federal prosecutor for the Northern District of Georgia who was now partner for the King & Spalding law firm.

Yates' résumé also includes stints as the US deputy attorney general under President Obama and acting attorney general under President

CHAPTER 8

Trump. She made headlines when Trump dismissed her for not filing arguments in defense of his refusal to allow travel, immigration and refugees from Muslim countries, his self-proclaimed "Muslim ban." She revealed her objections during congressional testimony by explaining the unlawfulness of the order, which Trump addressed in two subsequent revisions that added non-Muslim countries to the list. She also revealed her unwillingness to compromise character in the face of political pressure.

The Yates report is publicly available and is formerly known as "Report of the Independent Investigation to the U.S. Soccer Federation Concerning Allegations of Abusive Behavior and Sexual Misconduct in Women's Professional Soccer."[3] Her investigative team was composed entirely of women and included former federal prosecutors and college athletes, necessities given the legal investigative nature of the report and the witness sensitivities. The team was also incredibly well qualified, possessing both the technical expertise for the job and the personal connectivity to garner trust. Their charge was broad, to investigate both isolated incidents of abuse and sexual misconduct as well as "organizational awareness" or how a team, for example, acted or didn't act when abuses were reported. It was also limited in focus yet investigators pursued allegations and reports outside of the NWSL whenever it contributed to their principal mission. This included youth soccer.

Most of the report documents abuses committed by just three coaches, Paul Riley, Rory Dames and Christy Holly, and spans much of their careers extending into youth soccer. It is at times disturbing and graphic as it depicts a multi-faceted "culture of abuse, silence, and fear of retaliation [that] perpetuated the misconduct." The well-documented institutional apathy and tolerance reflects the systemic nature of the problem and at times, even during the investigation, involved deliberate interference, delay tactics and coverups by team and league management. Reviewing the entire study serves little purpose here other than to emphasize one key finding: "abuse in the NWSL is rooted in a deeper culture in women's soccer, beginning in youth leagues, that normalizes verbally abusive coaching and blurs boundaries between coaches and players."

Some of the coaches investigated had histories in youth soccer littered with abuse allegations. The more lurid accusations included inappropriate sexual relationships and even assault. For these coaches, training environments were often sexualized and grooming of both youth and professional players was evident. Verbal abuse or "tirades" were especially common if not expected. Players reported habituating to it and when combined with the blurring of player-coach relationships, players reported difficulty in distinguishing right from wrong behavior. They had grown so accustomed to being abused as youth athletes that they expected it as professional athletes.

The parallels between abuses documented in the NWSL and youth soccer were uncanny. They were also similarly rooted in a failed infrastructure. In the NWSL, the different organizations lacked appropriate player protections and established mechanisms or venues for reporting abuses. When confronted with abuse allegations, teams and the league failed to properly investigate and often rewarded the abuser. Those accused would frequently move to different teams with lavish press releases to whitewash records of abuse. Organizational leaders as well as those in the Federation were reported to have "privately acknowledged" the need for protections, yet for some reason they reacted instead of acted. The same can be said for the top leagues and teams in the DMV and, based on others' writings and investigations, across the country as well. Mechanisms exist for removing an unruly parent or spectator but not for policing coaches or even dealing with controversies. On my children's teams, there were no league, club or team mechanisms for confronting an abuser or bully or for reconciling controversies other than talking to the coach. But what if the coach was the problem? What if both coaches and the team manager were the problem? What, specifically, if all three modeled unprofessional, authoritarian and often childish behavior, creating an abusive environment where athletes and some parents openly ridiculed and victimized other athletes?

Our experience with the Coyotes, with the monothematic focus on winning at the expense of human development and, in particular, with the toxic patriarchal training environment, typifies the worst aspects of youth soccer and its especially corrosive effects on young women. Simply put, our Coyotes experience was a microcosm for all that can be bad in youth sports and especially in girls' soccer.

CHAPTER 8

Hyde's incessant berating and humiliating insults were complemented by Jekyll's enabling complacency. Witnesses to the madness, parents and players alike, reciprocated in kind as bully begat bully, predictably. Indeed, the entire team dynamic exemplified the classic bullying cycle with "bully-only" coaches and parents, "bully-victim" players and "victim-only" former players who either chose not to participate or who were cut from the team. These are clinical terms mind you, each with subgroups and unique risk profiles for negative and pathological outcomes that are surprisingly worst among bully-victims. These people are victimized by bullies and respond by becoming bullies themselves. They generally display the worst negative outcomes among the group and often suffer from serious psychological disorders. Anxiety and depression as well as rage, revenge, reward and recreational aggression are common, for example, while bully-victims are also more prone to weapon carrying, suicidal ideation and non-suicidal self-injury. Such outcomes aren't guaranteed, of course, and they vary in frequency and severity with the heterogeneity of subgroups. The medical community, nevertheless, rightly classifies bullying as a major public health problem with short- and long-term consequences affecting education and overall health.

The study of bullying specifically in youth sports is unfortunately an emerging field offering few if any sport-specific conclusions. Notwithstanding, bullying in sports is known to occur less frequently than in non-sports settings. Studies have also demonstrated sports participation to moderate bullying's deleterious effects, unless of course bullying infiltrates the playing environment via coaches who are bully-only participants, coaches complacent to bullying or those who overemphasize aggressive play, all of which occurred with the Coyotes. Overemphasizing aggressive play can blur the line between aggression and anger, which is already difficult for children and adolescents to distinguish. In fact, this cycle of aggression and confused anger is known to self-replicate and infect other athletes as it contributes to the bullying cycle.

"Nellie Oleson" was the team's aggressor and most notorious bully-victim. She openly bragged of her dirty and violent play and seemed proud to consciously and regularly cross moral lines, physically yet cleverly assaulting opponents as well as the Coyotes she despised. She was also the source of humiliating and insulting rumors spread by the "bully coven," a small group that often coordinated to harass other Coyotes. Most of the girls had habituated to the torment, although some parents later told me that the coven's and especially Nellie's bullying contributed to their daughters' bouts of depression.

Mei was Nellie's preferred target. From the very beginning, Nellie would menacingly stare at Mei throughout practice and, along with her familiar and team manager's daughter, "Veruca Salt," refused to pass Mei the ball in games. Coincidentally and consistent with the bully-victim profile, Nellie also experienced panic attacks and according to the girls may have struggled academically, two insecurities with potential to explain her malevolence but certainly not excuse it. Parents were all very well aware of Nellie's reputation and her parents even joked about it. I can only assume they tolerated her antics as an accepted cost of success because she was arguably the team's MVP, excluding Diana, although she was also a constant polarizing source of division and antagonism that limited not only team cohesiveness but also on-field success.

The rivalry with Mei peaked one evening after Nellie and Veruca harassed Mei continuously through practice. Every time Mei touched the ball, during drills or the scrimmage, they'd yell insults and personal attacks. The less inflammatory comments were masked as criticisms: "Why'd you pass to her . . . don't shoot, you weren't open." Many were obvious attempts to intimidate and humiliate: "God you suck! . . . I hate her." And some, said more softly and for Mei's ears only, were too rude to repeat. It didn't matter whether they were defending Mei or on the same team, standing next to her or 50 meters away. If you're a college basketball fan you know exactly what I'm describing, only this was more insidious.

Jekyll had stopped play toward the end of the scrimmage and was talking to the team. Most everyone was listening to him, except for Nellie who was standing next to Mei and had started whispering insults. When play began, Mei threw a well-placed elbow into Nellie's ribs, causing Nellie to briefly fall to the ground. Nellie then charged and shoved Mei from behind and after some colorful language, creative insults and artful posturing, the "fight" was broken up, not by Jekyll who did nothing but by the other girls. Mei came home seething in anger and hatred, vowing revenge on Nellie and Veruca and to punish the coven.

Chapter 8

Jekyll incredulously denied any knowledge of the incident. He also refused to intervene in what he belittled as "team politics" and discredited any responsibility for mentoring the girls. I was furious and demanded he protect my daughter as well as the coven's other targets. The team's dynamic had devolved into a feminine *Lord of the Flies* that could be parsed even by race with "the blondes"—their label not mine—in one group and the Latina, black, Jewish and mixed Asian girls in the other. The self-segregation was stark and obvious, in practice and infamously on a Boca Raton beach where the blondes demanded separate pictures, not all, but loudly and publicly. When I first heard one girl scream "only the blondes, only the blondes" I must have looked shocked because the mother of a black player said to me laughingly, "Did you really expect something different?"

I kept Mei home from the next practice. She was still very angry and not in a good place mentally. She despised Nellie and Veruca and I was honestly concerned that someone could get hurt. She also felt betrayed by her teammates' initial silence and understandably mistook it for partnering with the devil until four of them, all minorities, texted messages of support. The blondes remained silent and, in my opinion, complacent to the bullying.

It's easy in today's environment of oversensitivity to excuse some of this behavior to racism. After all, many of the coven's targets were racial minorities and the coven itself was composed of mostly blonde-haired white girls. Putting aside Occam's razor, however, the race angle is a little too convenient and honestly isn't supported by the fact that other minorities weren't bullied. I know these parents well and never saw any evidence of racism or support for extremist ideology. In fact, I'd describe almost every parent in the group as progressively liberal, some even radically liberal, and self-proclaimed champions of civil liberties and social awareness. Their tolerance for clearly race-based segregation, physical and emotional bullying and, probably worst of all, abusive patriarchal coaching makes them hypocrites, not evil, and like most of us, flawed.

The implied racial overtones were nevertheless legitimate. They were also upsetting to many parents of the non-blondes and were frequent topics of conversation for us, as was the bullying, derogatory and abusive language from the girls and the coaches, Hyde in particular. Mei once counted 12 consecutive F-bombs yelled at our goalie for making a bad play, not in an isolated practice or in a game with meaning, but in a friendly. It was a wholly unnecessary public shaming of a 13-year-old minority girl by a grown white man. She stood petrified in the goal, the two staring at each other as Hyde screamed from the sideline, "FUCK, FUCK, FUCK, FUCK, FUCK, FUCK, FUCK, FUCK, FUCK, FUCK, FUCK, FUCK!"

If you're appalled, imagine how the barely adolescent goalie felt.

Neither Jekyll nor Hyde had any grasp of the Holy Trinity. Both were master teachers of their trade and game managers. They were also adept at developing elite players, but at the expense of others with similar if not better potential. Even worse, they were utterly disinterested in mentoring, either through example or interaction, and were incapable of managing the emotional complexities of preadolescent and adolescent girls or even the expected jealousies of their parents. Hyde had once arrogantly told me that he had never met a parent who understood how to be objective. Until that moment, he had never met someone who actually taught a course on objectivity, "Science as a Way of Knowing," to top-tier undergraduate honors students. I doubt he was humbled by my mic-drop because it had little effect outside the conversation and both he and Jekyll continued to mismanage team dynamics, refuse all aspects of mentoring and remain susceptible to select influences.

This is of course my opinion, one that is shared by other Coyote players and parents, but not all. What isn't debated, however, is their legendary on-field antics that drew complaints from opposing teams and parents, from our own dysfunctional soccer family, from referees and officials, naturally, and even from strangers on neighboring fields. After we left the team, the family of a former 2005 Coyote purchased the house across the street from ours. Their daughter had grown tired of constantly being degraded and of Hyde's confrontational insults. Moreover, the parents were particularly concerned with the subliminal messages and precedent set by allowing a white man to verbally assault and intimidate their minority daughter so they too moved to a different team. Another minority and close friend from the 2006 Coyotes left at about the same

Chapter 8

time, after one of Hyde's tirades resulted in the girl's father being physically restrained for Hyde's protection. The world shrunk even smaller when we learned our other neighbor from across the street, literally next door to the 2005 Coyote family, pulled their son from Hyde's team many years earlier and for the same reason: verbal abuse.

My last straw came with Hyde publicly berating my daughter. She had been in the game for less than a minute and lost the ball on a physical challenge. She then pursued the girl for quite a long distance before returning to her rightful position. Play stopped shortly after and Hyde immediately replaced her, screaming insults and criticisms before she left the field, something he hadn't done the dozens of times other girls lost possession in the game. Her jog off the field turned into canter, a walk and then a crawl as she approached him; you could see the apprehension in her face and in her stance.

Mei had to leave the game early that day so I was waiting by the field's exit, standing 10 or 12 yards away from them with a fence separating us. Hyde wasn't bothered by Mei losing the ball but was beside himself with her "giving up" on the chase. She tried to explain that Jekyll had specifically instructed the team when and where to stop a pursuit, literally just days before, and was calmly and confidently explaining her position while Hyde was loudly and vociferously interrupting. At some point he shouted, ". . . STUPID." I honestly can't remember exactly what was said, "That's stupid . . . ," "Don't be stupid . . . ," "You're stupid . . . ," "Jekyll isn't that stupid . . . ," but the implication was undeniable. My daughter is stupid.

Several days passed before I could talk to Hyde, and he of course denied saying anything derogatory. He didn't apologize, feigning complete innocence even when I told him I heard every word. He was a hammer and the girls were nails. Jekyll was unwilling to intervene and I was beyond being patient. I saw the look of despair in Mei's face and the potential for a good yet challenging experience to sour completely. She was at a threshold, surviving the physical challenges of the sport, excelling at the athletic and overcoming the emotional, all to have the coaches pull the rug out from under her. It wasn't fair, it was abuse.

Mei unfortunately refused to quit the team. She was motivated by revenge, by the joy of beating the coven in practice and by her well-earned roll and successes on the pitch, yet her patience for Hyde's tirades were exhausted. I was resolute to change the dynamic and after many conversations with the Rush national leadership and then with the club directors, Hyde resigned and moved to another club. I have no idea if my complaints in turn precipitated his departure and if they did, whether he was asked or forced to resign, whether my pressure was his personal straw of contention or if it was all just coincidental timing. Nevertheless, he left and for a short time life on the Coyotes was pleasant, that is until he started poaching his favorite 2005 and 2006 players away to his new club. This ultimately precipitated the team's demise as players disbanded to multiple clubs throughout the DMV. Veruca's father experienced an existential crisis when she wasn't invited to Hyde's club and ridiculously threatened civil suits against Coyote parents all because Nellie's mother, the team treasurer, had the audacity to reimburse parents when the team disbanded.

In the end, the Coyotes were killed not by the competition but by the self-destructing influence of poor management. Specifically, by abusive authoritarian coaching and the resulting toxic byproducts. I appreciate Rush management for rightly intervening and wish I had contacted them sooner, although I question the motivation of local officials who were well aware of our coaches' antics and who didn't act until national leaders were involved. The local organization was managed almost entirely by men as only a couple girls' team coaches were women while all of the organizational leaders were men. The Coyotes were similarly "managed" by men and I've always wondered if the teams' hyper-masculinized and outdated authoritarian culture would have been tolerated if more women were in charge.

Hensley-Clancy explores a similar patriarchal culture in girls youth soccer at a population rather than personal scale in another *Washington Post* article that chronicles an environment best described as toxic to women and manipulative to girls.[4] It discusses sexism, sexual harassment and sexual assault throughout girls youth soccer, citing lawsuits at top ECNL clubs. It describes, quite ironically, an institutionalized boys club where highly experienced women are given menial tasks or low-level coaching assignments like kindergarten classes, where inexperienced men are assigned directorships and high-level teams. Bullying is also common as, for example, when women are routinely assigned the worst fields, disrespected and disparaged in meetings and forced to tolerate lewd and crude behavior, which appears to be the norm. Her reporting also suggests that clubs are frequently inhospitable to maternity leave requests and to the licensing needed for promotions, setting roadblocks by requiring women to play against men where they are physically bullied. She also discusses notable examples of inexperienced men being promoted without licensing over experienced and properly licensed women.

When the article was written, 90% of ECNL coaching directors, which is often the only full-time job in a club, and 85% of girls club directors were men. Approximately half of the clubs employed no women head coaches and many of the top clubs had no female employees whatsoever. The lack of any significant female influences in a girls' league is shocking and, from a civil court perspective, suggestive of illegal sexual discrimination. Moreover, the meager numbers hardly provide girls with proper role models or mentors capable of navigating or even understanding a girl's personal challenges. In my own experiences coaching high school track, I've had girls panic over their first menses, bleeding through their uniform. Others struggled with weight gain from oral contraception and with harassment from ex-boyfriends. I was lucky to have Mei and other older girls on the team who helped mentor and advise by proxy and, in a racially charged incident, a black head coach who could intervene in a way that only that demographic could respect. Club soccer teams are parsed by age and almost always coached by just one or two coaches who are usually white men so similar opportunities rarely exist.

Representation and role models matter, they really do, and with 70% of NWSL players having roots in the ECNL, a league dominated, controlled, managed and coached predominantly by men and in an environment plagued with sexual discrimination and harassment, where the athletes are commonly subjected to verbal abuse and misconduct as independently verified by multiple sources and investigations, is it any wonder that NWSL players as well as our daughters might be preconditioned to abuse?

The house cleaning that occurred in the NWSL after Linehan's article needs to occur in girls youth soccer. Many more women need to be appointed to leadership roles and to be offered advancement opportunities equivalent to men if not greater. These must include high-profile coaching assignments as the best players, those with the best opportunities to continue playing in college and professionally, are at greater risk for future abuses and thus require conditioning to recognize and respond to it. The goal should be to improve the training environment and development experience for our girls, and before this can happen women must first assume leadership roles. This includes within individual clubs and in high-profile leagues like the ECNL, EDP, Girls Academy, US Youth Soccer and the Olympic Development Program.

Lastly, every club and every league should do the following:

1. Establish an independently monitored website for anonymous reporting of abuse and misconduct.

   Children and parents need a safe mechanism for reporting suspected abuses or even voicing complaints that won't compromise their relationships with coaches or club administrators. This could even alleviate some organizational liability concerns by documenting allegations and responses.

2. Establish an independent review board composed of parents and community leaders unaffiliated with the organization.

   Boards would review reports of abuse, whether from known or anonymous sources, and make necessary recommendations to administrators or legal authorities like, for example, the police or child protective services. Guidelines for board action could be easily developed from those currently guiding school and other public entities. Note that independence is key and ensures that decisions are made objectively and without biased interference from coaches, parents or club/league administrators. Boards could even be shared between entities or tiered by team, club and league with relative independence depending on the local market size.

3. Adopt a Players' Bill of Rights built upon the ideals and rights proposed by the Aspen Institute's Children's Bill of Rights in Sports.

   Proposing a Bill of Rights or any code of conduct serves little purpose without the authority to enforce it. Thus, the bill should be used in annual reviews of any personnel who coach, mentor and/or advise a youth athlete. Such reviews are extremely common in business, government and academic sectors and are used to evaluate and track individual performance, reward successes and address deficits objectively. They're also used to ensure programmatic goals, which in this case is human and player development.

Such measures are almost always met with the same criticisms—they're cumbersome, they'll cost money, they'll never work—which in reality is nothing more than an expression of cost:benefit concerns. What do they cost in time, money and effort and what benefits can realistically be obtained? These are specious arguments at best, veiled knee-jerk reactions to oversight and regulation. The truth is that costs would be minimal, both in real and sweat equity, while the benefits to our daughters' health and safety would be invaluable.

Meilani's Take (17 Years Old)

Some of the best advice I ever received came from Jekyll: "I don't care what you have to do: scratch, shove, bite, just hurt her and get to that ball."

I'm kidding. That's horrible advice to tell an 11 year old. It's also typical of the team's "win by any means necessary" style of play, one that even condoned violence. Playing with the Coyotes was an *experience*, one that I'm happy to never relive. I'm grateful for it and I'm a better person and much better player because of it, but this doesn't excuse the abuse, belittling and Machiavellian play.

Jekyll was the principal coach for most of my first year with the Coyotes. He was strict and loud, occasionally obnoxious at games and was more sarcastic than insulting yet still intimidating. He'd irritate parents from other teams and many referees clearly despised him, but his antics and insults were trivial compared to Hyde's. As we got older,

Hyde began showing up to more practices, co-coaching more of our games, and before we knew it, he was calling all the shots. Jekyll's encouraging comments disappeared and were replaced by Hyde's verbal attacks. I remember preparing myself for practice, not strategically or mentally but emotionally. I remember the fear of being first in line where girls punctuated mistakes with a megaphone and Hyde would ridicule you, denigrating with nicknames like "dumb-dumb" for the day. Yes, he actually did this to me and loudly for all the girls to hear and maliciously repeat. I remember him yelling, "What are you, deaf? I said stop!" when I lapped the entire team during a conditioning drill. No appreciation for effort or accomplishment, just loud criticism as always. The joy of finishing first, of literally establishing my athletic dominance in an unprecedented beatdown was instantly lost and replaced with humiliation. I remember wanting to ask why he didn't criticize the slackers in the back for walking and cutting corners and chose instead to shame me for actually trying my best, but I knew, everyone on the team knew to never question Hyde.

My strongest emotional memory is of the stress and the caustic agitation in my stomach. I would feel it before most practices and it would get worse the closer I got to the field. When I first joined the team, practices were intimidating and when I eventually found my confidence, they became challenging often with cathartic rewards. They were rarely fun though and the prepractice agitation never disappeared. Other adjectives come to mind like irritating, frustrating and infuriating when I think about the bully coven, the coaches' absurdly biased favoritism and their lack of oversight as competition pitted girls against one another. Don't get me wrong, it wasn't all doom and gloom and I admit remembering the excitement and pride, not only from winning and scoring goals or even from the street cred I earned from playing on the team, but from receiving the rarest of gems, a coach's compliment.

Games were a conundrum. Playing and winning was of course exciting, but playing also presented opportunities to be humiliated. Every mistake like losing a challenge, diving in on the opponent's move or just not being in the right position could unleash a tirade of insults. "WHAT THE FUCK WAS THAT?" was always my favorite. It was embarrassing at first, but once I noticed the spectators' reactions, the look on their faces and how the other team's coaches would freeze in shock, it made me laugh. Abhorrent? Of course, but I had grown numb to it. I also don't think our coaches were oblivious to the reaction. I think they just didn't care or maybe they thought shouting profanity at a soccer game for 11 and 12 year olds, with their little sisters and brothers watching, was acceptable.

The Coyotes were ruled by fear. Fear of making a mistake, fear of failing, fear of disappointing the team and mostly fear of being humiliated. I honestly never feared losing because it rarely happened, but I admit the bench was often more inviting than the pitch. If the team played poorly, the tantrums could grow physical with coaches kicking coolers and tossing water bottles, hats or whatever else fell in their immediate sight. Their antics were notorious around the league and referees would say things like, "I've heard of you . . . Not you again . . . Oh, so you're the one . . ." They weren't the only children in charge and I saw many other coaches act this way especially in more competitive games and tournaments, but none so egregiously obnoxious as ours.

The girls relentlessly competed for our coaches' approval, especially Hyde's. We were attention hounds, always seeking the envy of our teammates. When my brother and I were young, my father would answer our annoyances with a question, "Do you want positive or negative attention?" and then follow it with a threat, "Because I'll give you negative attention!" It was a reminder that attention for attention's sake would not be rewarded. Most of the Coyotes carefully walked a similar razor's edge, never wanting to attract negative attention from the coaches but always playing for compliments. On the rare occasion that a small praise was expressed, joy was short lived because you were now the target of everyone on the team. It was an impossible task: playing for both the coaches' and teammates' approval. Such unhealthy competition was manifested in strange and unpredictable ways. Inside jokes about a player's faults spread among the cliques and clear favorites were picked from the bunch. Supposed "friends" would turn on each other simply because one received a "nice work" or similar innocuous compliment from a coach. It was such an ego boost! We had all been shamed on multiple occasions for making an insignificant mistake only to receive an unbalanced public castigation. Nobody was ever told to "run a lap" and mistakes were almost never missed. We also all quietly rejoiced when a teammate was rebuked whether or not it was deserved. I wasn't immune to this toxic trap and would brag at others' expense, we all did. It fueled personal growth at the expense of the team as well as my teammates' feelings.

My main issue was with the girls. I know the team's problems were actually rooted in coaching and in an atmosphere of animosity that nurtured unhealthy competition. The coaches were ultimately responsible. Some of the parents knew very well how their daughters behaved and shoulder some of the blame as well, but the girls themselves, some of them at least, were my tormentors. The struggle to maintain competitiveness—always—while also maintaining friendships was a constant strain on everyone. Some handled the strain better than others and some reveled and even took advantage of it. New players underwent a baptism by fire, never welcomed but hazed with glares, dirty fouls, constant whispers and behind-the-back giggles. We were fouling and hazing our own teammates.

The normal adolescent popularity game dominated team politics. Other than Nellie and Veruca, all the other girls were kind to my face. Even the bully coven could be nice, congratulating me on a goal or just goofing around between games, although I usually hung out with Arya and a couple other non-blondes. Arya was above the politics and was an intimidator. The bully coven feared her and our clique was usually ignored, which was fine with me. Backstabbing and rumors were common among the girls and everything was criticized, even the way a player dressed or didn't dress. Your shorts had to be rolled up at the waist, prewrap could only be worn on the edge of your forehead and braided high ponytails and Nike cleats were unofficially part of the official uniform. We even ridiculed other teams as trash players because they didn't meet our dress code standards. I'm embarrassed to admit it, but I freely participated in the charade of insecurities that were set by the select few and I distinctly remember shaming a person trying out because she had the audacity of wearing shorts that grazed the top of her knee.

Chapter 8

Despite the dysfunctions, the system was successful, successful in driving competitiveness, in creating championships and champion players and in attracting college recruiters to tournaments, but at what cost? Was all the toxicity necessary? Does winning really require vitriol, hate and animosity? I don't think so and I don't believe any of it justified our success. It instead reflects coaching weakness and a reliance on fear rather than knowledge, skill and maturity to lead the team. Some girls coped with the stress, others quit and some clearly struggled emotionally. I later learned that more than one was temporarily institutionalized from mental and emotional struggles that they attributed partly to the Coyotes. I mean, I doubt the Coyotes are completely to blame and my friends don't say as much, but the stress and bullying definitely made everything worse. My father would call this a "contributing factor." I call it messed up.

Looking back on the whole experience, I can't honestly say it was good, but I would be lying to say it was bad. It was like many things in life, nuanced and complicated. I met some of the worst people on that team but also formed close friendships. I was accurately described as "a deer in the headlights" aimlessly running around the field when I first joined but was promoted to playing up on the 2005 Coyote indoor futsal team after just one year. I was shamed and embarrassed by my coaches but also acquired a detailed knowledge of the game's ball skills, tactical approaches and psychology for winning. A central tenet to all of the world's moral philosophies and religions is that the ends never justify the means. But can they?

I've always been highly competitive. I would turn folding laundry into a race, homework into a tournament and Scrabble into a life-or-death fight, but the competitive nature of the Coyotes surpassed even my expectations and its toxicities left me wondering many times if joining the team was the right decision. After the night Nellie and I fought, I thought about this quietly on the entire ride home, not uttering a word until slamming the front door shut, collapsing on the stairs and tossing my cleats across the room. My father calmed me down, let me explain and with tears streaming down my red cheeks, not from fear or intimidation but anger and frustration, softly said, "We don't have to do this anymore."

My head shot up, "Absolutely not!"

I refused to allow a couple 12-year-old girls get to me. In no way were they better than me, not in soccer or in school and definitely not as teammates. I win, not them, and they would never intimidate or irritate me again. I showed up to practice with the same intensity I had before yet with a smile across my face. The nuisance girls were now targets and I dominated them like never before, openly taunting them at times and celebrating my victories in ways and words that are honestly a little embarrassing in hindsight. The entire experience left me with such mixed feelings. Not this specific incident or the unending taunting and backstabbing by Nellie, Veruca and the rest of the bully coven or even the abusive coaching but the entire Coyote experience. I appreciate and regret, and although elbowing Nellie, body shaming Veruca and throwing cheap fouls in practice doesn't reflect who I am as a person now or then but the circumstances that created it, I'd be lying if I said my retributions didn't feel wonderful. I'd also be lying if I didn't acknowledge the overwhelmingly positive effect it had on me. I'm a fighter with a stubborn, hard-headed never-surrender work ethic unafraid of challenge and I have the unhealthy Coyote experience to thank for it.

Chapter 9

Mount Rushmore

ANSON DORRANCE, HEAD COACH, UNIVERSITY OF NORTH CAROLINA WOMEN'S SOCCER
To say that Anson Dorrance belongs to an elite group of coaches is both cliché and inaccurate. He's elite of the elite. He's also hardly a household name even among the most ardent sports fans or for that matter soccer fans, likely because of the double sin of coaching a heretical women's sport. If I asked you to name the best college basketball or football coaches of all time or to create a Mount Rushmore of college coaches, several names would quickly come to mind, so many that you'd probably start debating the question itself. What did I mean by "best"? How should total wins, winning percentage and championships be prioritized? Should all coaches be considered or just NCAA Division I coaches?

John Wooden and Mike Krzyzewski would probably top most people's basketball list, Bear Bryant, Nick Saban and Knute Rockne atop football's, although I'm sure a healthy debate would follow any proclaimed champion. There would be no such debate when considering women's soccer. Anson Dorrance is not only the best and most successful coach in the sport's history, by any measure he's among the best regardless of sport, sex, division or era and would be my top pick for our Mount Rushmore of college coaches alongside John McDonnell (Arkansas, men's track and field/cross-country), Dan Gable (Iowa, wrestling) and Geno Auriemma (UConn, women's basketball).

Chapter 9

As of 2023, Dorrance has been coaching collegiate soccer for 47 years, 46 years as head coach at the University of North Carolina. He also coached the US Women's National Team for 9 years, winning the inaugural FIFA Women's World Cup in 1991 while still coaching at North Carolina. He actually began coaching North Carolina's men's team in 1977 and coached both the men's and women's teams for 10 years starting in 1979, which ended in 1989 when he focused solely on the women's team.

His record of accomplishment is unheralded and littered with firsts. He's the first in wins with 1,192 and an overall efficiency of about 90%, the first in Atlantic Coast Conference regular season and tournament championships with 23 and 22, respectively, and the first in national championships with 22. When the NCAA refused to organize a women's national championship, he partnered with the Association for Intercollegiate Athletics for Women or "AIAW" to organize the first collegiate soccer championship for women, which he won. The NCAA got their act together the following year and Dorrance again won. In fact, his women won 12 of the first 13 NCAA Division I national championships, 9 consecutively, a run exceeded only by UCLA men's basketball (10), LSU women's outdoor track and field (11) and Arkansas men's indoor track and field (12).

As the men's coach, his record of wins, losses and draws is 175–65–21 for a 70.8 winning percentage. He also won the conference championship in 1987 as well as the NCAA Coach of the Year award, his first of seven that are complemented by 12 such conference awards. He belongs to several different halls of soccer fame, has authored two books and a podcast series and has been featured in dozens of other similar publications. His ear and voice are highly sought and it was a privilege to interview him.

I asked questions about recruiting and skills development, about his training style and about coaching philosophies in general. The dialogue meandered between overlapping topics so rather than categorizing questions and answers, I've paraphrased his responses to the topical questions here. Mentoring served as a unifying thread, tying together myriad topics related to the development of youth athletes, the college athlete experience and specifically to his program. To my surprise, I learned that the foundation of his program rests on mental preparedness and not athletic fitness or specific soccer skillsets, which contrasts with every coach in my own and my children's experience. Advanced skills are of course desired and elite physical fitness was deemed a necessity, but maturity, coachability and what he described as "loving criticism" were paramount to his program and figured prominently when scouting potential recruits.

How do you evaluate talent?
Dorrance is a self-described slave to metrics and injects as much objectivity as possible into what is an inherently subjective process. He was speaking my language.

For example, each of his 30 players is ranked using 1-v-1 dueling. The results are recorded and winning percentages are monitored over time and used to track development in quite possibly the most valuable skill for any soccer player: beating the person in front of you. The drill itself as well as the scoreboard both help to drive healthy interpersonal competition that directly translates to wins on the pitch; winning challenges leads to more possessions that produce more crosses that create more shots that generate more goals. Pretty simple. Fun is integral to the exercise as Dorrance believes that "fun feeds competition" and competitiveness, in Dorrance's opinion, is the most critical skill and important characteristic of an elite athlete.

Dueling is just part of a more comprehensive training and evaluation system that incorporates win percentages and other metrics in a rubric of 10 categories (see the list that follows) that Dorrance believes are fundament to elite performance. His storied program attracts the nation's best players, all of whom aspire to play professionally if not for the US national and Olympic teams, so performance is quantified using a rigorous scoring matrix based upon these lofty goals. Each player receives a grade for each category on a scale of 1 to 5 where 5.0 has the equivalency of a US women's national team player, 4.5 a professional player, 4.0 a UNC starter, 3.5 a UNC reserve, 3.0 a reserve player worthy of traveling with the UNC team and 2.0 a reserve who doesn't travel or play. Anyone below 2.0 is probably in trouble.

Chapter 9

1. Self-discipline
2. Competitive fire
3. Self-belief
4. Loves ball
5. Loves game (play)
6. Loves game (watch)
7. Grit
8. Coachability
9. Energizing
10. Connection

The first three categories are the most important, consistent with Dorrance's belief that competitiveness and its roots in self-discipline and self-belief are critical. He allows athletes to score themselves for self-belief, which is a genius way to build confidence or, from a coaching perspective, to identify overconfidence or uncertainty. The three loves are meant to quantify devotion and sound like highly subjective measures, which they are, but quantifying a subjective measure provides a means to track progress. The point isn't the absolute number but how that number changes over time.

Coachability reflects how well athletes respond to all facets of direction and mentorship while energizing is a measure of attitude. Dorrance wants his players to display positive jubilant energy or, as he explains, "piss and vinegar," which for the younger readers isn't offensive but an idiom from John Steinbeck's *The Grapes of Wrath*. The man is very well read.

Connection refers specifically to relationships with teammates, not with the coaching staff or with anyone outside the team but with the fellow patriots and comrades-in-arms. The point is to build the solidarity, cohesiveness and trust that's critical to any successful team endeavor, and although it's tempting to believe that such interactions grow organically, Dorrance explains that it too requires coaching. He's a self-described introvert, although you'd never know it, and expresses empathy for others who are similarly shy and spends much of his private interaction time encouraging them to step out of their self-limiting comfort zone.

The fact that he values connections at all and literally quantifies them resonates with me. The form even lists names of players who Dorrance believes are most connected to each player. This is very similar to a guidance document I developed for the Graduate School at Washington State University, *Mentoring Maps*. Both tools, the connections and maps, serve to solidify support networks for students working and studying in high-pressure environments. Whether you're a PhD student juggling qualifying exams, teaching responsibilities and the publish-or-perish world of academia or an undergraduate student juggling mid-term and final exams, practice and classroom responsibilities and the championship-or-bust world of NCAA Division I athletics, you can't do it alone. Everyone has a team and everyone needs a teammate. Building connections with those more skilled or more prepared, or those who just support you, will help everyone involved to succeed, whether in athletics, academics or life.

Scores for each category are then used to calculate an average score without weighting. This is a very important distinction as every category carries equal value. He may personally view self-discipline, competitive fire and self-belief as the most important, but they all share equal value in the overall score that he defines as the player's "personal narrative of truth." His ultimate assessment is tabulated on a two-page form beginning with a summary of "Core Values Peer Evaluation" and the player's academic record, reminding each of us that these are student athletes with needs and responsibilities very different from professionals. The form then documents the player's ranking in the "Competitive Cauldron," which includes the 1-v-1 and other drills, as well as rankings in athletic testing and technical testing of various soccer skills like serving the ball, shooting power and accuracy, proficiency with both feet and heading the ball.

Dorrance shares the form and his evaluations with his players at least three times a year in private meetings where they discuss their score and, as a result, their standing on the team, their progress and improvement and sometimes their regression. It's an exercise in objectivity and maturity and probably best illustrates "loving criticism."

Players are taught to appreciate criticism and to differentiate constructive from destructive criticism, although my impression is that this often occurs as trial by fire. He generalized the current generation of high school athletes as being uncharacteristically self-absorbed compared to previous generations, and in his defense I doubt few would object. This generation is far less likely to be given responsibilities even for themselves, to hold jobs outside of home or be told "no." That last one is a personal observation, but the others are very well documented. In fact, the employment rate of Gen Z'ers ages 15 to 17 is about 18% compared to 27% for Millennials at the same age and 41% for Gen X'ers, according to 2018 Pew Research data. The disparity continues among young adults ages 18 to 22 with 62%, 71% and 79%, respectively. This isn't necessarily bad, but it is real and it represents a legitimate training challenge. How do you get someone to accept responsibility for their teammates when they've never been responsible for themselves?

A key to this transition Dorrance believes is the team's Core Values. I've reproduced them here, word for word from the current version. They were originally penned in 2006 but have evolved slightly over the years, sometimes incorporating quotes from the likes of George Bernard Shaw, John Donne, contemporary writers and friends. Obscure symbols from obscure places and things, like the "careful cycle" symbol from washing machines and the Hittite cuneiform script for "king," have also been added. I haven't included these or most of the quotes because they're really just elegantly worded supplements. The last Core Value represents the most recent addition, a contribution by the team's 2018 Leadership Council, which is composed of senior players and one leader from each class. They advise Dorrance on issues with lasting importance, those extending beyond the scope of team captains. The value itself addresses a generational concern and greatly illustrates the plasticity of Dorrance's training and mentoring program.

1. *We don't whine.* This **tough** individual can handle any situation and never complains about anything on or off the field.
    "The true joy in life is to be a force of fortune instead of a feverish, selfish little clod of ailments and grievances complaining that the world will not devote itself to making you happy." George Bernard Shaw
2. *The truly extraordinary do something every day.* This individual has remarkable **self-discipline**, does the summer workout sheets from

beginning to end without omission or substitution, and every day has a plan to do something to get better.
3. *We want these four years of college to be rich, valuable and deep.* This is that **focused** individual that is here for the "right reason" to get an education. She leads her life here with the proper balance and an orientation towards her intellectual growth, and against the highest public standards and most noble universal ideals, she makes good choices to best represent herself, her team, and her university.
4. *We work hard.* This individual embodies the "indefatigable human spirit" and never stops pushing herself. She is absolutely **relentless** in training and in the match.
5. *We don't freak out over ridiculous issues or live in fragile states of emotional catharsis or create crises where none should exist.* The best example is the even-keeled stoic that is forever unflappable and **resilient**. The worst example is the "over-bred dog," that high maintenance, overly sensitive "flower" that becomes unstable or volatile over nothing significant.
6. *We choose to be positive.* Nothing can depress or upset this powerful and **positive** life force—no mood swings, not even negative circumstances can affect this "rock."
7. *We treat everyone with respect.* This is that **classy** angel that goes out of her way to never separate herself from anyone or make anyone feel beneath her.
8. *We care about each other as teammates and as human beings.* George Floyd, Breonna Taylor, Ahmaud Arbery, Sandra Bland and all other Black lives lost to police brutality, this "Bell Toll" has galvanized all of us to live this extraordinarily powerful and important core value. This is that non-judgmental, **caring** and inclusive friend that never says a negative thing about anyone and embraces everyone because of their humanity, with no elitist separation by academic class, social class, race, religious preference, or sexual orientation.
9. *When we don't play as much as we would like we are noble and still support the team and its mission.* This remarkably **noble**, self-sacrificing, generous human being always places the team before herself.

10. *We play for each other.* This is the kind of player that works herself to death covering for all of her teammates in the toughest games. Her effort and care (her verbal encouragement) make her a pleasure to play with and her **selflessness** on and off the field helps everyone around her.

    "People don't care how much you know until they know how much you care." Rakel Karvelsson, a former UNC player and member of the Iceland women's national football team, in a note given to Dorrance.
11. *We are well led.* (A) This is the verbal leader on the field that is less concerned about her popularity and more concerned about holding everyone to their highest standards and driving her teammates to their potential. This **galvanizing** person competes all the time and demands that everyone else do as well! (B) This is that leader who lives our core values and tries to get those around her to live them as well. She is not shy about calling people out who don't live them and not afraid to protect those not present when others are trashing them.
12. *We want our lives (and not just in soccer) to be never ending ascensions, but for that to happen properly our fundamental attitude about life and our appreciation for it is critical.* This is that humble, gracious high-achiever that is **grateful** for everything that she has been given in life, and has a contagious generosity and optimism that lights up a room just by walking into it.
13. *Accountable.* This is the biggest challenge for the Millenials. Now is the period to escape the protections of loving parents who don't want you to get hurt. You have four years to get ready for "the chaos of the universe." Marc Cohen, and award-winning UNC assistant professor of English and Comparative Literature, when asked "Who was the best teacher you ever had and why?" said this: "The best teacher I've ever had is Failure. Samuel Beckett said it best: 'Ever tried. Ever failed. No matter. Try again. Fail again. Fail better.'"

Dorrance also explains these values in an interview with Dr. John Silva, a UNC Professor of sport psychology in the Department of Exercise and Sport Science, where they discuss the psychology of coaching. The emphases on competitiveness and confidence are constantly addressed and Dorrance notes that building such traits requires distinctly different approaches with men and women. Screaming at players, for example, can motivate men but not women. "You can't lead women with your own personality. . . . That's totally ineffective with women. What happens when you are that way with a woman, unless you have a very good and close personal relationship with her is that you are going to actually shatter her confidence."

Dorrance's anecdotal accounts may sound a little sexist when read in a vacuum, but he's careful to admit his ignorance and suggests that both biological and social pressures are likely responsible for the sexual dimorphism he's noticed. You also can't argue with his success and with his emphasis on mentoring and the ability to be mentored, a point I know I'm belaboring but one that is clearly a foundation to programmatic success and elite player development.

What are the critical skills coaches look for when recruiting?

Dorrance doesn't believe in a scouting consensus and suggests that different coaches use different criteria to suit their specific needs. He further admits that it's nearly impossible to accurately evaluate recruits using his objective system and instead uses the good old "eye test" while being very mindful of the 10 categories.

"Fitness and fight" (i.e., competitiveness) he believes are most important while leadership is the "special sauce." Leadership can be difficult to evaluate with transient interactions at camps and I noticed he didn't define it with formalities like being captain of teams. He instead looks to see how players treat their teammates, whether they support the less talented, praise accomplishment and encourage the team or alternatively, if they're constantly critical, selfish and dismissive or, as he summed, "just jerks."

Dean Smith, the legendary and hall of fame UNC men's basketball coach with two NCAA national championships and the fifth most Division I wins, taught him to carefully watch how recruits interact with their parents. He believed that parent:child interactions were windows of character, and Dorrance confirmed that recruits who treated their parents with disrespect would similarly treat their teammates. Respectful kids, by contrast, were excellent teammates. In fact, parents and parenting came up several times during our discussions, in ways both positive and negative, although some of the malevolent and team-disrupting behaviors he's witnessed over the years, as well as those many of us have experienced, may just as likely have grown from indulgent coaching. After all, too much of any fertilizer will feed a weed.

Dorrance rarely recruits for a specific position and only when addressing a weakness. Goalie is the one exception as it requires not only skillsets unique to the position but also height and reach. Among position players who satisfy the eye test for fitness, fight and leadership, the advantage goes to versatility, which is far more valuable to Dorrance than demonstrated success at a given position. Non-goalies are generally classified as central or flank players. The former need to be physical and must head the ball well, flank players need to demonstrate speed, technique and vision while all players must demonstrate good decision making. This was the first and only time he mentioned specific traits in our discussion and you probably noticed the lack of specifics in his specifics. He never mentioned, for example, thresholds for running speed or endurance, timed cone drills or even exit velocity on kicks. Scoring or creating goals and especially winning duels with or against the dribble get him excited, and when I asked about his concerns, he sheepishly stated that a history of multiple injuries raises a red flag, which I interpreted as empathy on his part. He then said that a disqualifying trait is a bad attitude and teammate issues. This dogmatic conviction against recruiting prima donnas surprised me and overshadowed everything we discussed. It also flies in the face of most youth soccer coaches I've met who in my experience adopt an "end justifies the means" attitude.

What non-soccer credentials most interest you?
"Great academics, but it's rare."

A little-known secret among the academe is that UNC is one of the most respected public universities in the world. What it lacks in Nobel laureates and, as a result, general public street cred, it compensates for with rigor and selectivity, having admission rates comparable to more well-recognized peer institutions like the University of Michigan and the University of California, Berkeley. In fact, the US News & World Report ranks UNC as fifth overall among public universities with Berkeley and Michigan as first and third, respectively. In 2022, Berkeley admitted just 11% of applicants, 14% as California residents and just 7% from out of state, approximately 50% of which were international applicants. Both Michigan and UNC accepted about 20% overall and 40% from residents, but UNC accepted only 8% of non-residents versus 18% for Michigan.

Non-residents are held to higher standards with university admissions because the pot is only so big. Admission policies can be quite political and are often set legislatively. This includes non-resident quotas, and because there's less room for international and out-of-state students in the pot, the qualifications of those admitted—grades, standardized test scores and essays—are usually far better than those of in-state students. This means that the average NCAA Division I student athlete, who is already superior to 98% of other high school athletes, needs to also be academically superior to 92% of non-resident UNC applicants. Such students aren't unicorns, but they are exceedingly rare as is the likelihood that the average non-resident student athlete could compete for a prestigious academic scholarship.

From this perspective, Dorrance's program is a victim of its own success. He attracts athletes from across the globe, each of whom must compete for admission with some of the brightest young minds in the country. In fact, 22 of his current 29 players are non-resident students. He further admits that most of his non-resident recruits couldn't compete for academic scholarships and the few that have were truly Ivy-level students in the class room but generally not starters much less stand-out talents on the pitch. Filling his roster, therefore, requires exceptions to normal admission standards, which may be true for most Division I programs, but not to the same degree as at UNC. He and other coaches are dying for academically strong athletes, those who could attract academic scholarships and help spread the athletic scholarship wealth. His goal, however, and that of most universities is to maintain a minimal standard GPA, which at UNC means maintaining a 3.0 every semester.

Chapter 9

After discussing academics, Dorrance immediately returned to the "special sauce." I get the impression that leadership is always on his mind, as a topic and as a scouting trait, although he again rarely finds recruits with much special sauce at all. The topic clearly excites him and he admits to reading anything written by or about Winston Churchill, the quintessential 20th-century leader and savior of the British Isles. He also appears anxious to share opinions that could naively sound controversial.

He believes that good leadership qualities are hard to find in young women. Young women often don't display the same level of confidence as young men and are also more concerned with perceptions than with outcomes, unless of course perceptions are the desired outcome. His experiences coaching both men's and women's teams suggest that men are more apt to identify and resolve problems and to take the necessary initiative. In the interview with Silva, he even stated disbelief in the ability to make grand changes in leadership abilities despite the claims of self-help gurus: "I think we all land somewhere on the leadership continuum, and I think we can move someone along the continuum to a degree, but I don't think you can transform someone, the way leadership institutes feel they can."

Nevertheless, he isn't deterred and claims to devote substantial time to developing leaders on his team and leadership characteristics in all of his players, which I believe is reflected in the Core Values. This is a bit self-serving as he claims that he's lost with good teams that lacked leaders and won with bad teams, relatively speaking, with good leaders. Thus, it is indeed in his as well as the program's interest to identify leadership traits in his recruits or at least the potential to move the continuum. When I asked him to explain the underlying cause for such disparity between the sexes, he suggested that basic biology could play some significant role but felt that training and society are more responsible. He doesn't believe girls are given the same opportunities to lead on or off the pitch and that the patriarchal youth soccer system for girls is more than emblematic of the problem: it's partly and possibly largely responsible. We specifically discussed elite leagues like the Elite Clubs National League (ECNL) that have a predominance of male role models in coaching and he sees this as a major contributing hurdle. It teaches girls to follow rather than lead, especially to follow men, because girls almost never see women in leadership positions.

Lastly, he discussed "loving critics" and "loving criticism," a training ideology that he deeply embraces. It's the freedom to give and receive criticism without judgment—the essence of objectivity. It's founded on trust and develops slowly by building personal and team connections with private mentoring and with team exercises. Imagine how quickly and efficiently a coach could train a new technique or offensive scheme, for example, or how any teacher could overcome even the most complicated intellectual barriers if both teacher and student were unencumbered by the emotions of pride. Trust is the cornerstone so it's not surprising that finding a recruit with this skill is incredibly rare. After all, he hasn't had time to build the trust and I suspect the rarity is due to high school and club coaches not investing the effort and to the expected immaturity of adolescents. Notwithstanding, any recruit demonstrating "loving criticism" immediately attracts his attention.

What criteria do you use to evaluate the merits of a scholarship offer?
Dorrance began his answer by first explaining the numbers of recruiting. The university limits him to just seven incoming athletes, usually freshmen. The magic number was only five when the system pursued seniors and was expanded when colleges started recruiting high school freshmen. He estimates that one of the five exceeded the scouting report expectations, two were spot-on, one was worse than expected and one struggled to get even a modicum of playing time. This explains his self-proclaimed 60% "hit rate" on identifying quality players as three of five met or exceeded his expectations. His hit rate dropped significantly when colleges started to recruit younger athletes, which he attributes to the nearly impossible challenge of accurately evaluating the athletic and emotional potential of a 14 year old. The university eventually allowed him to expand his recruiting class to seven and as a result, restored his estimated 60% hit rate.

NCAA Division I regulations allow each women's soccer team to provide 14 scholarships, which Dorrance distributes among his 30 rostered athletes. Roughly 6 to 8 receive full scholarships, 12 to 14 receive partial scholarships and the remaining 10 are classified as "walk-ons" and play without scholarship. Dorrance quickly pointed out that most of these latter students would likely have never met the university's rigid admission standards without his support. Their benefit is, therefore, two-fold as they're exposed to world-class coaching and a world-class education, both of which couldn't have happened without soccer.

As for the specific criteria, he returned to the Core Values, the Competitive Cauldron and what he described as the means to achieving his personal narrative to truth: "loving critics." The man is consistent.

Do you have any concerns with youth soccer?
"Yes, kids are quitting in droves around the ages of 14 to 16."

Dorrance attributes the loss to burnout. He also believes that parents and coaches are equally culpable in creating the performance pressure that drives kids away from the sport. He referred me to the three loves—of the ball, of the game and of watching soccer—and suggested that pressure is counterintuitive to developing love of anything and can actually drive children in the opposite direction. He didn't use the word "hate," but that was the essence of his point.

This was the only time in the interview that I initially disagreed with Dorrance, not that the loss of youth players is a problem or that pressure per se could be the underlying cause or even that coaches and training environments are contributors. We've both formed our opinions from our own anecdotal experiences in the youth soccer arena and both are subject to relative bias. I interact mostly with concerned parents who blame coaches as blood sport for all of their children's woes. He interacts mostly with coaches who conveniently excuse every player dysfunction on poor parenting. I suspect our opinions are to a degree both flawed and correct and admit that I've seen many instances of parental pressure crossing the moral line. However, I've also seen abhorrent behavior from coaches, and so has Dorrance, as well as disinterest and incompetence that could similarly compromise the love.

In the end, I was swayed by his argument. There is no single point of blame. This is why Dorrance strongly criticizes the misdirected overemphasis on *player* development instead of *human* development, a sin committed by parents and coaches alike. Mentorship, the molding of character, and the emphasis on fun as the hook or buy-in to a demanding training environment are integral to his program. They're enablers of trust, to loving criticism, to the team's core values and, as a result, to championships. Parents and coaches take note.

ID or showcase, training video or game footage, YouTube or subscription services—what do you like to see in a player biography and how should they present themselves?
"ID camp is great!"

Dorrance designs his identification or "ID" camps to mimic a typical UNC training environment. Athletes of course perform basic drills to assess basic skills, but this is a minor component of the program. Competition features prominently in the itinerary with 1-v-1, 5-v-5 and 11-v-11 games and as I've witnessed each for myself, they can be intense. His ID camps are proving grounds for UNC hopefuls, whether or not they're legitimate contenders, and for athletes with lower or just different aspirations. Most importantly, they provide an opportunity for close personal evaluations of a few targeted recruits.

It's important to understand the distinction between ID camps and summer or day camps. The latter are usually much less competitive. They provide a revenue stream for collegiate programs so the vast majority of campers will never receive a serious look from any of the coaching staff and when they do, the staff are so well trained that they can quickly categorize campers into "here for the experience" and "maybe she's got something" pools. Mind you these are my words, an attempt to paraphrase his sentiments, although he readily admits that only a very select few attract his attention at summer camps. He adds the caveat, however, that the truly elite will always get noticed, whether at summer or ID camps, showcases or tournaments; talent—like cream—will always rise to the top.

ID camps are programmatic investments. Breaking even financially would be cause to celebrate, the proverbial icing on the cake where cake is identifying or successfully landing a top-tier recruit. Registration fees for ID camps support non-salaried staff as well as necessities like sport drink and medical supplies. The leftovers pay for swag like tee shirts, water bottles or drawstring bags, all emblazoned with university or team branding. Such goodies often pale in comparison to day camp swag and for good reason: ID camps are all business.

Dorrance couldn't emphasize enough the importance of repeated exposure, not within a given or short period of time, as in a single season or even over a year, but as the athlete transitions from a youth to adult player. Continuity, consistency, growth and improvement can't be measured acutely, only with repeated if not chronic observation, and in a perfect world, Dorrance would see the same athletes every year starting in middle school. As I discuss, puberty alone can enhance or deter athletic development in young women who often become slower with less endurance capacity, yet stronger and with training, more skilled. Thus, it's not uncommon for an athlete to suddenly improve in one or many facets of her game or to compensate for a weakness. This underscores the importance of repeated exposure especially with top programs like UNC that regularly recruit freshmen.

He only briefly discussed showcases, noting that it's interesting to evaluate in a team-versus-team environment, which he also does *ad nauseam* at ID camps. However, he didn't go into detail when discussing showcases and used ambiguous terms like "sometimes," "often" and "can" rather than absolute terms like "definite" and "best" when describing the benefits. I'm again paraphrasing, but he specifically stated that the quality of evaluations in a showcase depends upon the quality of the teams involved and later admitted that "a combination [of ID camps and showcases] are best, but even summer camps are good." He further admitted to enjoying highlight videos, but he felt his and his staff's personal evaluations were far more valuable to the process.

It's important to pay attention to the adjectives and descriptive terms Dorrance uses if one is to decipher his preferences and priorities. For example, he describes ID camps as "great," showcases as "wonderful," summer camps as "good" and videos as "nice." The key, I believe, is his trust in personal evaluations.

***Last thoughts, is there anything you want
players, parents or coaches to know?***
His advice to players: "There are two simple things to add to your regular training sessions to be extraordinary: live on a wall and play 1-v-1 to win."

He defined "living on a wall" as literally shooting against a wall, with both legs as hard and often as possible. He felt this was the most efficient use of personal practice time as it helps to develop power with both feet while recovering the rebound helps develop the first touch. He also noted that a short session on the wall will easily surpass the number of touches a starter would experience in a typical game that, according to his data, results in just three to four minutes of actual ball handling. He recognizes the tedium of the wall drill, however, and that most young players lack the patience needed to reap the rewards, a challenge for any task dependent upon delayed gratification. He then begged the questions, "Do you have the discipline to live on the wall? Do you have the love?"

He next emphasized winning on both sides of the ball when playing 1-v-1, consistent with his infatuation with competitiveness. In his experience, girls are far less likely to voluntarily play confrontational games like 1-v-1 and will instead play turn-taking or team games. Some examples from my daughter include "world cup," a group game synonymous to basketball's "knock-out" or "bump"; "Swedish fish," where teams of two compete in shooting and blocking goals; and "nothing but net" or "cross bar," self-explanatory games based on their namesake. Dorrance believes that mastering 1-v-1 is crucial to mastering the game and is quite possibly the most important skill. This is why he urges girls to challenge themselves, to overcome whatever insecurities or perceptions that limit their development. He wants them to embrace confrontation, to lean in figuratively and literally, and play 1-v-1 as much and as often as possible. I couldn't help notice that he again focused on the very fundamental physical and mental traits of the game: shoot hard, control the ball and fight like hell.

His advice to parents was more poignant, more critical and, for some, more difficult to hear: "Raising kids with an overwhelming personal narrative of unquestioned positivity is noble and may help to build self-esteem and confidence, but most people don't live with a true personal narrative." He further explained that narratives are constructed defensively, for protection and via means that I would describe as Darwinian. The parental focus on positivity can, therefore, morph into overindulgence and in the absence of constructive criticism can create a false narrative.

He criticizes this generation's parents for creating "participation trophy culture" free of criticism and children who are overly concerned with feelings instead of emotional maturity and character. He believes many kids are being raised without standards and that this shatters respect for authority. Psychologists have written volumes on the topic, political pundits have debated its social merits and comedians have ridiculed the generation with abandon so I see no need to beat the dead horse further. I'll note, however, that his training often shocks new players who are unaccustomed to critiques, uncomfortable with criticism and don't understand objectivity; the path to "loving critics" is getting longer with each generation.

I agree that this sounds a bit like conservative ideology. He assured me it's not and was characteristically honest in expressing contempt for the conservative insensitivities that plague our headlines, not conservatism per se as we never discussed politics but the attacks on people and the worshiping of negative stereotypes. My impression is that he embraces liberal ideological values regarding equality, acceptance and respect, but realistic and pragmatic ideologies of character. He makes direct comparisons to the parenting approaches I discuss in previous chapters without specifically naming them. I found his perspective refreshing even when critical because his philosophies and approach to coaching mirrored authori*tative* parenting. They were based on objectivity and transparency and rejected authori*tarian* and indulgent approaches. I applaud his desire for recruits to embrace self-responsibility and feel, as I hope you do as well, that everyone, this generation and beyond, would follow his advice.

Geno Auriemma, Head Coach, University of Connecticut Women's Basketball

Geno Auriemma isn't a household name, but it's close. Anyone following women's collegiate basketball, women's Olympic basketball, basketball in general, any competitive sport or aspect of contemporary American culture or anyone who's ever watched ESPN during the months of November through March since 1985 has heard of "Geno." His name is synonymous with "championship" and is as recognizable as "Coach K," "Brady," "Ali," "Lombardi" or any other sports legend.

This is one of two important distinctions between Auriemma and Dorrance and it's related to the other. Both coaches are cut from the same magical cloth of accomplishment and are rightly worthy of Mount Rushmore enshrinement. Like Dorrance, Auriemma ranks first in games coached, wins, winning percentage (>88%) and number of NCAA Championships. Both coaches lead in professional recognition in their sports: Auriemma with 8 Naismith, 9 Associated Press, 6 US Basketball Writers' Association, 10 conference as well as other coach of the year awards. In fact, the USBWA renamed their award to the "Geno Auriemma Award" in 2024. Both also coached US women's national teams winning Olympic and/or world championships.

Their personalities and coaching philosophies are identical, which probably isn't a surprise considering that they're of similar age and have been coaching a women's collegiate sport for nearly the same number of years, spanning identical decades and experiencing sea changes in NCAA regulations, university oversight, funding and sport popularity. Auriemma never had to create a national championship tournament out of thin air as Dorrance did. Then again, Dorrance's program isn't remotely impacted to the degree of Auriemma's by student name-image-likeness or "NIL" monetization issues. This is because women's collegiate and professional soccer, unlike basketball, is still mostly ignored by the national media. The Women's National Basketball Association (WNBA), for example, was the fastest growing brand in 2024 with 3.82% growth for all adults and was ranked 18th with women and 3rd with men.[1] Its games are regularly televised and league revenue tripled from 2022 to a whopping $200,000,000 in 2023.[2] Similar growth could potentially occur with women's soccer as according to the *FIFA Women's Football: Member Association Survey Report 2023*,[3] global participation in organized soccer for girls and women increased by approximately 25% since 2019, continuing along its meteoric rise. The US leads the world in participation with approximately 1.8 million adult women over the age of 20 playing in a registered league, and this is larger than the total number of female participants in all of Europe regardless of age.

The threshold for attracting media attention for most sports is established by successes in its professional franchises, and although an entire USWNT and four former players from the dominant 1990s USWNT have appeared on Wheaties boxes—the pinnacle of athletic success—not a single professional women's soccer player outside of our national teams has ever been similarly honored. Breakfast cereal aside, this brings us to the second and very important distinction between Auriemma and Dorrance: the NIL.

Allowing student athletes to financially benefit from their name, image and likeness is not only fair, it's consistent with several student-employee relationships in academia. Undergraduate work-study students, for example, get paid to perform menial to professional tasks on every campus in the country. The federal program provides stipends for part-time work and unlike student loans, they aren't repaid. One could argue that work-study students are nothing more than part-time employees with regulated hours and compensation, which they are. One could also make the same argument for graduate student research assistants and for college athletes. Graduate student teaching assistants receive full-tuition waivers in addition to a part-time stipend and, thanks to collective bargaining, health insurance. Moreover, graduate student research assistants, especially in science fields, receive the same benefits but often higher stipends than teaching assistants yet their research assignments—drum roll please—are their own research project!

The precedent for paying students to perform tasks that are unrelated or directly related to their education while also providing free tuition was established decades ago. Am I surprised it took universities so long to finally apply this well-worn model to the college athlete? No. I love academia and I'm its biggest defender, but to describe universities as miserly would be inaccurate; avaricious or money-grubbing would not.

NIL profoundly impacts the managing of athletic programs in ways only coaches of revenue-generating sports anticipated. Women's soccer generates no or almost no revenue on the vast majority of college campuses and even storied programs like North Carolina's must supplement ticket sales with summer camps, ID camps, special events and donor contributions all in a losing effort to break even, which they never do. On the other hand, UConn women's basketball program is the most visible collegiate program in the world, attracting talent from every corner of the globe and, from alumni and fans, high expectations. In 2023, the program generated the third-highest revenue on campus, $4.4 million (reported by Zaakirah Mujid, BVM Sports, February 22, 2024), behind men's basketball and football, yet it still wasn't self-supporting. In fact, no NCAA women's basketball program is self-supporting. Each is supplemented by donations and development and by money from the profit-generating sports: football and men's basketball. Revenue generating is a far cry from profitability or even revenue neutrality.

College athletics are not minor league programs. Universities, administrators and especially coaches are tasked with an education mission unparalleled by any professional system including development leagues like Major League Baseball's minor league system or the National Basketball Association's G-league, two stupendously successful professional mentoring systems that have never accounted for final exam schedules. The reality is that the cost of maintaining competitive and academic excellence in most collegiate programs far exceeds their typically paltry revenue stream. Graduation rates under Auriemma and Dorrance have traditionally beat their respective non-athlete campus rates as well as the national rates for their sport. They have also frequently reached 100%, including most recently in 2023, which is testament to their commitment and valuing of the student-athlete mission.

Auriemma's recruiting is clearly impacted by the NIL. The degree pales in comparison to that of high-profile men's sports, say for example UConn men's basketball or Ohio State University football, which paid an approximate total of $20 million in 2024 to their players (according to several news sources), but it permeates every aspect of recruiting and some of team management. It also ran as a common thread linking much of our discussion to what I learned is the reality of contemporary collegiate sports.

How do you evaluate talent?
"I don't," he quipped. "If a kid doesn't have enough talent, I'd never get the opportunity to see her."

Recruits are first identified by a network of "talent searchers" composed of assistant coaches who also serve as recruiters. NCAA rules were recently modified to allow six coaches, including head coaches, and four designated recruiters to participate in the process, one that is highly regulated with restrictions on how and when talent searchers can interact with potential recruits. He attempted to summarize and address it throughout the discussion, yet despite his best efforts I found it as disorienting as a concussion.

The entrance bar to his program is high and the select few that survive the recruiters' critique are then advanced to Auriemma who primarily evaluates the recruits' non-basketball credentials. He, like Dorrance, is interested in the team player, one willing to sacrifice self-interest for the greater good of the team. Is the player unselfish? How does she handle bad calls or being taken out of the game? Does she celebrate and prioritize team or individual successes? Is she about the *me* or the *we*?

His next question surprised me, introspectively. "How do their parents behave in the stands?"

He believes that many parents, not all or even most but a significant amount to warrant concern, disregard these traits. He insists that many misunderstand the goal, which should be to support their child and to ensure a joyful playing experience while molding their character. This is the true goal of competitive athletics, he insists, not scholarships or NIL money. I mentioned my love of Tolstoy's *Three Questions* and he appreciated the analogous comparison to his own coaching and mentoring philosophy.

Some parents, he continued, try too hard to live a second life through their child's experiences, a mistake he admits to making himself and one that I too have made. He then asked, "Are they coached or encouraged at home?" The answer, he believes, is often a telltale sign of maturity and an important determinant in making recruiting decisions.

What are the critical skills coaches look for when recruiting?
"Typical offensive skills."

He then explained that most coaches emphasize overall athletic ability as the sport demands competence in a variety of skillsets and in physical fitness. Skill level or specialization in a particular skill as, for example, shooting from distance, passing or rebounding, or even size and speed are valued differently depending on a program's needs and coaches' playing style, but good offensive skills are a litmus for most. Top-tier programs like his insist on sound fundamentals across the board. Meeting this criterium, however, functions as a go/no-go, a binary checkpoint for concluding or continuing the evaluation, which as he emphasized was heavily influenced by non-basketball credentials.

What non-basketball credentials most interest you?
Character, character, character! This isn't a direct quote, but it could have been.

Auriemma looks for unselfish interactions with teammates, both on and off the court. He wants athletes who are easy to coach, who respond to objective criticism responsibly instead of defensively, those who encourage and thrive with it and who are accountable as much for their mistakes as they are with their triumphs. He admits to playing favorites, but not in the way most parents or players suspect. His favorites *aren't*. They *aren't* the best or most gifted athletes. They *aren't* the top scorer or best defender. Most importantly, they *aren't* a "pain in the ass." They are instead repulsed by drama and are committed to the team with a laser focus on winning.

They are also good students. He insists that academic potential is reflected in character and notes that "95% of college athletes are terrific students with good academics. They study on the plane, show up to study hall every day [and are] accountable." Laziness, he insists, is the primary reason some student athletes struggle with academics. "Ninety percent of my kids fit a profile of strong character and upbringing." When I asked about the other 10%, he responded, "Most of time the kid is great, but the situation isn't."

He then explained how the transfer portal—a relatively new mechanism to help students move between programs without losing eligibility—has helped resolve irreconcilable differences that, in the past, could fester at a team's expense. Athletes intent on leaving had to choose between sacrificing a year of eligibility or leaving school for an entire academic year. "Coaches can [now] tell a kid you can't play here anymore and they leave willingly."

He wanted to emphasize how much support the average student athlete receives, noting that in addition to scholarships and athletic training, they receive academic support, healthcare, counseling, mentorship, "everything," yet they often leave if they're not played. He never wants an athlete to leave and I got the impression that he considers it a personal failure, at least to some degree. The few who have left did so amicably he believes and that the decision was mutual albeit sometimes painful. The discussions are always difficult and some athletes choose to stay despite concerns over playing time. This often presents a new challenge to Auriemma and his coaching staff, not with the athlete but with parents unwilling to accept the reality of their child's independence and, in many instances, with FERPA (Family Educational Rights and Privacy Act) regulations that prevent any university official from discussing academic issues with anyone other than the student.

FERPA is also known as the Buckley Amendment. It protects student educational records that are broadly defined as "all records maintained by the institution." Ambiguity aside, it ensures confidentiality with very few exceptions for specific and legally defined situations. Once a student becomes a legal adult, FERPA protected rights transfer from parent to student and although discussions of playing time per se aren't protected by FERPA, discussing why playing time is being restricted, the underlying academic and personal problems, very often are. This is why Auriemma admits to ignoring parents in these situations and rightly focuses on managing the student athlete's needs.

I've been in the same situation myself, with undergraduate academic advisees clinging to medical or veterinary school aspirations despite having an abysmal GPA or with graduate students reconciling their underestimated assumptions with the reality of graduate school rigor. It's difficult on everyone and as a parent I sympathize with the desire to intervene, but Auriemma and other caring coaches are not only legally but morally justified in prioritizing the rights of student athletes over their parents' insecurities.

Auriemma's message to parents is simple. Teach your child to be responsible, for themselves, for the team and, of course, for their grades. He preaches responsibility and I gather is unaccepting of excuses. He also claims little credit for his athletes' successes and believes that good coaches provide only the opportunity to succeed. They find joy in helping kids—their athletes—transition into adulthood, which involves winning and losing, challenges on the court and in the classroom as well as struggles in their personal life. If this sounds like a recipe for mentoring, it is. In fact, he talked very little about basketball, the game or the skills, and constantly brought up character. This dominated the conversation in many ways and in a lighthearted way I would accuse him of being obsessed with it.

"Coaches *should* be mentors," he insisted, "and the vast majority of them are totally invested in their kids." I'm not sure I agree with "vast majority" and have written *ad nauseam* about how some coach for themselves and about the systemic abuses in girls' and womens' soccer, but this isn't my nor Auriemma's point. He believes that coaching young athletes, which includes college athletes, is vastly different from coaching adults. Youth and college coaches are obligated to mentor, and although he didn't explicitly describe those who don't as failures, he did describe the failure to mentor as a failure to coach.

"In the late 80s, coaches were everything," he explained. "You didn't just recruit a kid, you adopted them whereas today you're just one of many voices in their head. Social media, parents, family and friends and even professional sports agents [are all advising on] brand. It's a *huge* distraction. Some handle it like a pro, others really don't at all."

CHAPTER 9

His job as coach and mentor has apparently gotten harder to do and I suspect this explains why he values character so very much. He considers it integral to personal, athletic and academic success, and from a pragmatic perspective, recruiting for it makes his job just a little easier.

How many scholarships are you allocated, how are they typically distributed and what criteria do you use to evaluate the merits of an offer?
Auriemma explained that the NCAA allows universities to provide 15 total scholarships to a Division I basketball program and unlike some sports, they can't be parsed among athletes. This differs significantly from Dorrance's program and from collegiate soccer in general where fewer scholarships, 14 at UNC, are often distributed in full or in part among 30 or more athletes. Auriemma suspects the NCAA will eventually end scholarship parsing for all sports. He didn't predict the impact, although his tone was skeptical if not negative and he admitted that he only wants or needs 12. He also described recruiting walk-ons in most of his previous years and, like Dorrance, emphasized their importance to team dynamics as much as to success.

Universities and the NCAA prefer that basketball teams receive 15 scholarships because this helps balance Title IX requirements that mandate equal protection under the law. Until 1972, discriminatory funding of men's and women's athletics was legally allowed and universities generally funded revenue-generating men's sports and ignored women's. Title IX of the 1972 Education Amendments act was intentionally modeled after Title VI of the 1964 Civil Rights Act and ended such discriminatory practices.

> *No person in the United States shall, on the basis of sex, be excluded from participation in, be denied the benefits of, or be subjected to discrimination under any education program or activity receiving Federal financial assistance.*

Universities are swimming in federal supplements so to stay compliant, they reluctantly provided athletic scholarships to women. It's important to note that non-revenue-generating men's sports were receiving scholarships at the time so there really was no logical objection. In the years since passing Title IX, men's teams have occasionally been sacrificed to maintain a particular university's compliance, although the overall goal of supporting parity in education—and student athletes are indeed students—has been preserved equally between the sexes, although not necessarily between sports. Why does a basketball program receive 15 scholarships to support 100% of its athletes when soccer receives 14 to support just 40 to 50%?

Demographics are unlikely to explain the disparity as although minority representation in basketball is typically higher than soccer at most universities, track and field, which also has a typical minority representation that exceeds soccer, must also parse scholarships. Auriemma didn't comment on this and I suspect he would be in hot water if he did, but he did describe the average scholarship athlete as being "super-compensated." Moreover, he expressed empathy and respect for walk-ons and the average student working through school who similarly struggle to balance the challenges of academic with non-academic responsibilities.

"I support the NIL at every level, but some kids expect $100,000. Some kids have agents in high school and there's nothing wrong with that, but this ability to work with agents creates *have* and *have-nots* among schools." I'll add to different programs as well. Among the *haves* is of course UConn women's basketball and his expression of empathy reflects, in my opinion, concern over an imperfect system in flux, one where confusion reigns and the role of contemporary college coaches has forever changed. Scholarship decisions must no longer consider talent, fit and need alone, but also affordability as *value*—in defining a recruit's potential—has adopted an altogether different meaning.

Do you have any concerns with youth basketball?
Yes, coaching! Again, not a quote, but it could have been.

He references youth soccer in Europe as a successful modern system that requires licensing and formal training of coaches. This is in stark contrast to youth sports in the United States where licensing is generally encouraged but not officially required for most sports. When it occurs, it's generally informal and unregulated with rare oversight or accountability. He believes teams are diluted by "sub-par coaching" and that quality coaching in youth basketball is rare. His opinions perfectly align with the Children's Bill of Rights in Sports that, if the reader remembers, emphasizes mentoring over winning and calls for formal training and licensing.

"Coaching is very difficult. The most important characteristic kids need to learn is how to be on a team, that the universe doesn't revolve around you because life is about being on teams. . . . Whether you're on the playground, at work or school, or with your family, you're never alone. Working together is extremely important."

ID or showcase, training video or game footage, YouTube or subscription services—what do you like to see in a player biography and how should they present themselves?
Auriemma distrusts highlight films and describes them as misleading. He sees value in videos of entire games where he can watch players perform on and off the ball and in the context of team play, but he emphasized that even this pales in comparison to witnessing a recruit perform in person. He no longer runs basketball camps, however, and was quite emphatic in describing why. Parents would drop off approximately 500 kids a week, his estimate, with little interest in formal basketball training. It was probably a valuable public service and generated a little revenue, but running a basketball-focused childcare, my words, didn't help to evaluate talent. Something like the tiered system that Dorrance created to funnel legitimate recruits into separate ID camps or that isolates better athletes into "maybe she's got something" pools may be a necessity for most non-revenue-generating sports, but not for UConn women's basketball.

Top-tier programs like UConn's attract the best of the best. Their challenge isn't finding the talent but finding and scheduling opportunities to watch and assess the talent. Showcase events and tournaments are common venues for these purposes, and Auriemma admits to using recruiting service lists to find when and where potential recruits are playing.

These services arose from a recruiting process that most non-college coaches would consider unnecessarily complex and its befuddling effects have fueled rapid growth of an industry that didn't exist when I was in high school. Companies like the obtusely named Next College Student Athlete (NCSA), which is the self-touted largest recruiting platform and was founded in 2000, and SportsRecruits (2008) are among the better recognized. If awarded an NCAA certification, they can list their subscribed football and basketball players on the NCAA website, although I assume most companies aren't certified because very few of their websites actually advertise it. NCSA, for example, devotes an entire webpage to "NCAA Certification and Compliance" whereas it isn't mentioned on the SportsRecruits site and possibly the oldest company, National Scouting Report (1980), devotes a page to explaining why they choose not to certify. Remember that certification only applies to football and basketball and listing services aren't offered for other sports. This dilutes the influence of most recruiting services companies to little more than website hosts.

The NCSA site is possibly the best developed and provides resources explaining the recruiting process and NCAA regulations, advice on getting noticed and a platform for coaches and athletes to connect with video uploads and player statistics. It's important to realize that these for-profit companies are in no way endorsed by Auriemma, Dorrance or me and that they are only associated with the NCAA through the listing service. In fact, even the NCAA describes "approval" with quotations, which I interpret as distancing if not somehow invalidating the certification process itself.

The services provide value to parents and athletes, but they aren't invaluable in any way, and according to Auriemma and many other coaches I've interviewed, coaches use them with varying and questionable degrees. Auriemma trusts only his and his team's evaluations and admits to only using the services for location purposes. He also questions how parents use it to "advertise" their kids, a criticism commonly expressed by many coaches. In other words, mine to be specific, it's a system for *selling* rather than *evaluating*.

CHAPTER 9

Last thoughts, is there anything you want players, parents or coaches to know?

He answered immediately, "Do you know Jannik Sinner, the Italian tennis player? His parents let him leave home at 13 to go to school and live on his own, to make his own decisions without his parents' influence. This gave him the independence and confidence to make decisions." Auriemma continued, referring to parallels in a youth hockey system that allows kids to play away from home, free from parental concern, pressure and criticism, all of which I respected but also questioned. I certainly wasn't willing to relinquish my children's safety, education, character and emotional development to an athletic pedagogue and I'll risk betting that the vast majority of readers feel likewise, but this wasn't his point.

Auriemma is concerned that parents pressure kids far too much. That their own unfulfilled dreams masked in the most common excuse, the quest for a Division 1 scholarship, or a new and more sinister excuse, an NIL windfall, compromises their better judgment. To paraphrase an idiom from this book, he's concerned with *parents parenting for themselves and not for their kids*, a mistake he and I readily admit we've made ourselves.

Letting go is difficult for every parent, but it's necessary and it should probably be done earlier than most of us admit, and this is Auriemma's point.

Finally, I asked about his training program, whether it was as structured as Dorrance's with, for example, quantifiable rubrics and core values. He laughed and admitted to similarly adopting a set of core values, but didn't elaborate, and an emphasis on character, competition and teamwork. He then said, "Anson's way smarter than me, we don't do that," and again laughed. He was being cheekily obtuse, but I didn't pursue it further. He clearly has a system and it's clearly successful. Its details, however, were in his mind and for the purpose of this book, inconsequential to his take home message. Person before player, the rest will follow.

Chapter 10

Plot Twists

Poor Oedipus. The original star-crossed victim of tragedy was destined to infamy by the Oracle of Delphi, Pythia, an old lady with a direct line to Apollo, the Greek god of sun and light, music and poetry. Pythia foretold Oedipus' murder of his own father and his incestuous marriage to his mother and, as is common of most mythological stories, fate cannot be denied. Oedipus flees his adopted parents' home in Corinth and in an incident of Greco-Roman road rage, he unknowingly and accidently slays his true biological father before continuing on to Thebes where he eventually marries Jocosta, again unknowing that she is actually his biological mother. Although Pythia's prophecy is fulfilled in stages, Oedipus' acceptance comes suddenly, when he learns that his newborn son is also his brother. Jocosta hangs herself and poor Oedipus gouges out his eyes, a fitful punishment for arrogantly tempting one's fate and challenging the will and wrath of gods.

Sophocles' use of peripeteia in *Oedipus Rex* is typical of Greek tragedies, indeed of many tragedies. This literary device, pronounced "per-*uh*-pi-**tahy**-uh" or "-**tee**-*uh*," is used to shock or stun the reader with a precipitous plot change followed by negative or tragic consequences and reversals of fortune. Think of it as a eureka moment of doom. This contrasts with the predictability of dramatic crescendos and creates jaw-dropping moments and literal gasps. A slightly more recent example of peripeteia can be found in *Million Dollar Baby*, a movie starring Hilary

Chapter 10

Swank, Morgan Freeman and Clint Eastwood, who also directed. It tells a story of a female boxer, Maggie Fitzgerald, who is similarly star crossed and reminds us that the consequences for tempting fate, whether with Greek or boxing gods, is tragic.

The Sixth Sense, by contrast, uses *deus ex machina* for similar but not identical effect. Pronounced "dā-ə eks mä-**ki**-nə," this Greek saying translates to English as "a god from a machine" where "machine" refers to the mechanical device used to suspend flying characters above ancient Greek or Roman stages. The literary device differs from peripeteia by producing positive rather than tragic consequences. Think of it as a eureka moment of salvation. This occurs when Dr. Malcom Crowe, played by Bruce Willis, suddenly realizes why he is so uniquely qualified to help 9-year-old Cole Sear, played by Haley Joel Osment, end his torment by New England's apparitions and poltergeists.

Classical antiquities they're not and neither movie make my list of top-five all-time best (see chapter 7) or even come close to it, but they're very entertaining and provide excellent modern examples of peripeteia and *deus ex machina* and how these tools bridge exultation with gloom and conflict with resolution, respectively. Probably more significant is that they define limits of existentialism. Fate was a supersonic cruise missile in *Oedipus Rex* and *Million Dollar Baby*, stealthily approaching at unfathomable speeds until impact. No decision could have prevented Oedipus' or Maggie's tragedies. In *The Sixth Sense*, fate is merely a puzzle that disappears once solved, providing peaceful resolution to both Sear and Crowe.

Youth athletes all too often experience sudden and precipitous change brought on most often by injury, although not always. Academic, family, health or social challenges or any other unforeseeable catastrophe can derail the path to Division I stardom or even varsity playing time whether or not said event is truly catastrophic. After all, timing is everything in the recruiting world so any setback in high school can disrupt the recruiting process, especially as many athletes start receiving serious looks in their sophomore and sometimes freshman years and establish verbal commitments in their junior year. Whether such events exemplify peripeteia or *deus ex machina* are somewhat fate dependent, although I'd argue that the long-term consequences are entirely subject to existentialism. Only you can decide whether to gouge out your eyes or, alternatively, to follow the Marine Corps moto: improvise, adapt and overcome.

Mei faced many challenges as a youth athlete. Some common, others serious, and in every instance, she improvised, adapted and overcame. I'm very proud of her resilience and mental fortitude and strongly believe she'd make an excellent Marine. She even considered applying to the Naval Academy and has visited the campus many times, running on the indoor and outdoor tracks and taking an official tour, which I highly recommend to everyone. She possesses the composure of a fighter pilot, the focus of a sniper and the fealty of, well, a Marine, but her aptitude is better suited for a courtroom than a battlefield. She indeed has mettle. It was forged through competition, on pitches and tracks, in front of white boards and debate judges, with blood and sweat but never tears and despite climatic severities that exemplified peripeteia, existentialism prevailed, she prevailed.

She's lived a life of privilege, not by race or attitude, but by stability in family, income and education. She's never needed and although all children want, she was taught the value of "no" at an early age and has always appreciated the difference. She has nevertheless experienced a greater share of challenges than I believe fate would demand. The common were to some degree social, as with the bully coven, and at times with subjective coaching, as with Jekyll and Hyde, but they were all chronic irritations at worst and although injuries were prevalent, most resolved quickly with physical therapy and hard work. Like I said, Mei always prevails. Her story, however, is truly tragic, not comparatively as I'll explain, but from the perspective of an elite adolescent athlete, is worthy of Shakespearean respect.

Act I: Exposition and Incident
By the time the Coyotes dissolved, Mei was playing and running at top form. She was highly accomplished in two sports having qualified for the indoor and outdoor USATF and AAU National Track Championships many times in addition to playing for one of the nation's best soccer teams. The Coyotes' fate was drifting powerless due to Hyde's departure

for a rival club and to many parents quietly debating the merits of jumping ship. Several team meetings had been held, initially to quell concerns over Jekyll's new role as the sole coach and later to dispel rumors of the team's demise, although to stick with the nautical metaphor the Coyotes were listing and rats were fleeing quickly. In just a few weeks, the once-storied Coyotes were reduced to a single player, Veruca, and to her father who filled former parents' inboxes with pathetic legal threats to recoup refunded fees. It was a sad and well-deserved ending to a club with arguably unmatched potential ruined by mismanagement.

Mei was at a crossroads. Should she specialize in just one sport or continue with both? If just one, which? If both, how?

It wasn't an easy decision, and as a parent I felt obligated to help, to guide her decision and to provide any assistance, information or resource available. I offered to hire private coaches, to train her myself or to coordinate practices with school, club and private coaches. I offered to drive her throughout the DMV and up and down I-95 chasing distant clubs, meets and tournaments. I naturally offered my opinion, free of judgment, influence or bias, all within reason, and it was a mistake. All of it was a monumental mistake in parenting. The advice was sound, the offers were sincere and my intent was laudable, but they were also all mistakes.

Mei was 14 at the time and perfectly capable of making responsible choices. Her opinions are frustratingly well articulated at times and she's never been afraid of sharing. My mistake wasn't in respecting her choice or her opinion or even her process. My mistake was in not respecting her. I failed to realize that my opinion as a father, as one of the two guiding mentors in her life and the absolutely most significant influencer of her youth athletic career, could overshadow her own. When I needed to be silent, I spoke. When I needed to retreat, I approached and when I needed to just let it be, I acted. I loved, but I didn't respect.

She/I decided to continue with both sports, but to prioritize track. She had always been tiny and although her speed, endurance and technical skills allowed her to compete with other elite soccer players, her size was a detriment and she had been injured many times because of it. She had grown aggressive, possibly too aggressive, playing with the Coyotes and had experienced three ankle sprains. Nothing too serious, but each required weeks of physical therapy. I reasoned that the probability of serious future injury was significantly higher playing soccer and that her best opportunities to compete in college would be on the track and not the pitch. Thus, we looked for a suitable competitive soccer club, hired a private track coach and committed to playing and running for her high school teams, all while pursuing a highly competitive advanced placement curriculum in school, maintaining a perfect GPA and competing in debate and *a cappella*. It was definitely too much, but she agreed that academics were her top priority and that soccer could be sacrificed if needed.

The COVID-19 pandemic had delayed the spring club soccer season as well as high school track. Mei was a freshman and spent most of her time outside of class running with her private track coach and occasionally juggling a soccer ball. Practices, meets, tournaments and league games eventually returned and by the soccer season's midpoint, Mei led her new ECNL team in goals and assists while playing as an outside forward. The team itself was a far cry from the Coyotes, lacking both talent and drive and until Mei, another former Coyote and a couple girls from other ECNL teams joined, had never won a tournament. They lacked focus and commitment and their laziness often frustrated their coach, Nancy Rohrman, and the new players, but the overall experience was stress free and pleasureful. Nancy welcomed Mei's two-sport commitment and, true to her word, never criticized when track meets or practices conflicted with her soccer schedule. She referred to Mei as her "go-to girl" and understood what many parents and some youth coaches often don't, that every player is unique with issues and challenges that often require specific and sometimes specialized management. The girls were having fun, collecting laughs, wins and an occasional trophy. Club soccer was once again enjoyable.

Track, by contrast, had begun inauspiciously despite training privately with arguably the best private coach in the Mid-Atlantic. Kris Jost had won national championships as a distance runner in high school and for Villanova University where she won multiple All-American and All-Academic awards. She had also coached high school track and cross-country for many years, winning state championships and, at the storied Bullis High School, some national championships. She understood

Chapter 10

the intricacies of training adolescent girls in particular and had placed many of her athletes in highly prestigious collegiate programs. She's eccentric and jovial, bordering on odd with a volcanic enthusiasm that overshadows even that of her athletes. Despite being an education major in college, her understanding of exercise physiology far exceeds any high school or club coach I've ever met, regardless of sport. My only criticism of Kris is that we shared the gift of gab and were compatible to the point of being incompatible: our conversations would drone on endlessly, often to Mei's ire.

The pandemic was still a concern and only outdoor sports were allowed. This meant that the winter indoor track season would be canceled, but fall high school soccer could continue with a restricted season. Kris started to build Mei's base focusing on long and threshold runs. The latter help the body clear lactic acid from muscles and enable athletes to run fast frequently or over long distances, which would benefit soccer and middle-distance runners equally. Mei was only a freshman yet worked her way into a starting role as the right winger for the varsity team. She was still tiny and very skinny, but her speed and ability to cover the field tirelessly impressed her coach; Kris' workouts and Mei's work ethic were paying dividends.

Mei practiced primarily outdoors, often running or playing in the cold Mid-Atlantic rain and sleet and occasionally during a snow. She sometimes ran at the Naval Academy's indoor facility but had developed a mild case of exercise-induced asthma that was exacerbated by dry air. Running indoors was especially difficult and she experienced her first serious attack in a Virginia Beach facility where, ironically, a commonly prescribed and usually effective beta-agonist, albuterol, completely failed. Her bronchioles constricted after 600 meters into an 800-meter race and she struggled to complete the final lap, wheezing and collapsing at the finish.

I was immediately engulfed by a sense of fear and guilt. Fear from the natural protective reaction every parent would feel watching their child suffer, a feeling quashed to some degree by a medical understanding of the risks playing out before my eyes, and guilt from my conscious and unconscious influences over her decision. We were less than a year into "The Plan" and I was already questioning it.

Kris had experience managing runners with exercise-induced asthma and with a motherly instinct calmed Mei down before giving her a nebulizer. This is critically important because the rapid short breathing pattern would prevent albuterol from reaching the target depths of the lungs. Kris was unique in this regard, the only coach in Mei's youth athletic career with such experience, which contrasted greatly with her high school track coach, "Noz," a recent college graduate with little experience as a coach, no knowledge of training distance, middle-distance or high performing athletes with asthma. Moreover, he was adamantly opposed to collaborative coaching and demanded Mei quit either the high school team or private training. The school athletic director thankfully intervened, allowing Mei's workload to be managed by Kris and me as Noz ignored her.

Coach Noz's reluctance to coordinate training with Kris is not atypical of high school track and cross-country coaches in our area and I suspect at large. According to several local club coaches, the aversion to co-coaching is actually the norm. A multitude of factors likely contribute and although dysfunctional personalities and sensitive egos may play a role, the track culture itself is probably more to blame. After all, participation in club team sports like soccer, baseball, basketball and lacrosse is extremely high throughout the DMV, but not for track and field or cross-country. The clubs that do exist provide incredible opportunities for young athletes, but almost all of them stop participating once they matriculate to high school where team sports operate within a culture of competing club opportunities that simply don't exist for track. This is purely hypothetical, but I suspect the naïveté of most high school track coaches contributes to an adversarial rather than collaborative approach to co-coaching. They either fail to see the advantage of an athlete gaining elite experiences in elite venues and instead focus on potential complications and risks that are, in my opinion, lazy excuses for inaction, or they're coaching for themselves.

Anyone unfamiliar with youth club sports will be surprised by how significantly superior it is to the average high school experience. I certainly was. I also assumed the mixing of age groups and the selection process inherent to large school varsity programs would combine to

Chapter 10

produce a superior product, but I was wrong. High school teams operate on a restricted schedule and with athletes of assorted skills whereas clubs practice year-round and with athletes that often specialize at early ages and as a result have accumulated a tsunami of experience that easily overwhelms mismatched athletes who play primarily or exclusively for their schools. This means that high school teams with more club players or with more players from better clubs usually win.

Most of the former 2005 and 2006 Coyotes attended public and private high schools in our area. Mei was the only former Coyote to play for Thomas S. Wootton whereas their rival, Walt Whitman High School, rostered six and were favored to win multiple state championships. Mei would only play two years, however, as "The Plan" gradually weaned her off soccer, initially by moving to a less competitive club team and then to replacing high school soccer with cross-country. Wootton won nearly every game during Mei's tenure, a cathartic string of victories over every team with a former Coyote. The only loss came during a state tournament rematch against Whitman who scored the winning goal in the last 10 seconds of the second overtime. Mei blanketed the field, dropping on defense and isolating one of the state's best forwards, a former Coyote and vitriolic member of the bully coven. Mei stole the ball from her multiple times, functionally benching her from the game, all on an ankle pieced together with prewrap, athletic tape and ibuprofen.

I watched her hobble off the field with the Whitman girls jumping and cheering in the background. She stopped to hug a close friend and one of Wootton's elite players who had torn her anterior cruciate ligament, the infamous "ACL" injury, in the last few seconds of the last regular season game. She was a senior, watching from the sidelines and leaning on crutches as her and Mei's only chance to experience a state championship vaporized in a flash.

Mei had ironically sprained her ankle on a threshold run with three other girls training under Kris' guidance. They had reached the halfway point in an out-and-back run along the Potomac River and switched positions, running fast with only a single step separating the two-by-two rows. Threshold runs are long and fast and are run at 85 to 90% of maximum heart rate. They're uncomfortably comfortable, difficult in the beginning and painful in the end.

Mei led on the way out and had switched to the back row after the turnaround. She had found the zone and was pushing hard, focusing on her friend's heels, taking care not to clip them. The girls were running in sync with the precision of a military march, but much faster. Left heel, right heel, left heel, right heel—concentrating helps forget the pain—left heel, right heel, left heel, right heel, walnut.

Mei was on her back in an instant. She described an audible pop—ligaments snapping—and piercing pain that was all too familiar. She had sprained her ankle once again.

I ran that morning as well, in the opposite direction from the girls, and was surprised by beating them back to the parking lot. The trail was littered with walnuts still encased in their husks, some the size of baseballs and all hard as marble and heavy. You could hear them crashing through leaves and hitting the ground with a heavy thud. We ironically referred to them as "ankle-breakers."

I continued running after a few minutes and eventually found Mei a mile and a half from the lot. Her ankle was badly inflamed with swelling pushing up her leg. She couldn't bend or walk on it and was using her friend as a substitute crutch. I then carried Mei back to the car, alternating between piggy-back, my shoulders and sack-o-potatoes. She vetoed fireman's carry.

Imaging confirmed what we already knew was a severe low ankle sprain. The orthopedist immobilized the ankle with a boot and prescribed standard RICE therapy, an anti-inflammatory and physical therapy. The latter worked miracles and quickly restored range of motion, flexibility and torque around the joint. It also prevented lower limb muscle atrophy, all of which saved her soccer season.

Her ankle issues were always concerning and when we were finally able to walk away from soccer, I was relieved. Every challenge on the pitch made me nervous and every tackle made me gasp. I still felt apprehension at track meets, but injury was never a concern. I instead worried whether she'd get trapped inside, if she'd hit her splits and about baton exchanges.

Chapter 10

Worries over children never disappear but pivot, change and morph as they age. When Mei was an infant, I'd wake every night, lick my palm and place it under her nose to ensure she was breathing. My wife celebrated her sleeping through the night whereas I struggled adapting from the 3:00 a.m. feed and would wake instead for the life check. With track, I worried about overtraining and nutrition. She was running over 40 miles a week with long, high-intensity interval and threshold runs and would struggle to maintain weight. Thus, I worried about bone mineralization, amenorrhea and self-esteem, although the worry *du jour* was asthma and it was steadily getting worse.

Mei struggled through the indoor track season her sophomore year. Breathing was difficult when running high-intensity intervals and she mostly wheezed when competing. We experimented with different drugs and treatment regimens and eventually settled on a combinatory drug, Symbicort, that includes an inhaled long-acting beta-agonist (formoterol) as well as a corticosteroid (budesonide). This carried her through summer training and over a promising fall cross-country season but was again ineffective running indoors. No distance or middle-distance runners, especially, enjoy running indoors and frequently complain about "dome lungs," all except Mei who couldn't find the breath to complain. She tried better hydration schemes, sucking throat lozenges and altered Symbicort doses and regimens, yet nothing worked. It was a season of wheezing and disappointed finishes.

"The Plan" was always on my mind and so was the guilt. It wasn't too late to switch back to soccer so I sat her down and devised a backup, "The Plan 2.0." She assured me that she preferred track and that she wanted to run in college. She had bested her 800m PR by one second during her outdoor sophomore year and was intent on breaking 2:15, the recognized threshold time for Division I scholarships. She's also a pragmatist and admitted that the lack of progress was discouraging and agreed that soccer might be a better option if she couldn't at least break 2:20.

Her best that season was 2:23, set in a 4x800-meter relay. She struggled to breathe in every race, often finishing seven or eight seconds slower with times she had smashed three years earlier. It was time to initiate "The Plan 2.0."

Mei was still reluctant and I didn't want to force a decision, but one had to be made. We discussed the pros and cons of continuing to focus exclusively on track, assuming her asthma stabilized. I would gladly support a return to her true love, soccer, and would even support her participating in both sports if we could devise a schedule that didn't compromise her academics or exacerbate her asthma. Mei was still unsure, anchored by an obligation to her cross-country coach. She had been voted captain and didn't want to disappoint the coach or team. I was proud of her commitment, loyalty and maturity and in a way her willingness to self-sacrifice for the greater good but finally decided to end the nonsense when she admitted to hating track.

"What do you mean you 'hate track'!"

I was shocked, not that a child would hate running mile after mile in the rain and snow or sprinting endless high-intensity intervals with negligible rest under the blazing heat of a sweaty Mid-Atlantic bug-filled summer. I was shocked that a child would do such torturous things and pretend to like it.

"Why didn't you tell me? Why torture yourself? Why weren't you honest, with me and yourself?" I asked, although they were more demands for answers than questions.

"Because I was good at it."

Children want to please. They want to please their friends and siblings. They want to please their teachers and coaches and they desperately want to please their parents, so much that they'll sacrifice themselves for the attention, respect and love that they instinctually crave. Child psychologists recognize that this behavior changes with development and wanes with self-assertiveness and independence. Mei has always asserted herself and has never shied from any opportunity to go it alone yet, I suspect, her commitment to the sport of track and the unparalleled demands of distance and middle-distance running were rooted in the Darwinian act of pleasing Dada. Maybe not entirely and definitely not in adolescence, but how much of her more recent devotion can be attributed to inertia? How much did I consciously or unconsciously influence her?

Chapter 10

Overwhelmed with guilt, I changed the conversation from "What is best" to "What do *you* want to do?" I urged her to be honest, to hold nothing back, to . . .

"I want to play soccer. I love soccer, I always have, I'm good at it too and I think I can play in college."

"Do you really want to play in college?" I asked.

"Maybe, if it's Berkeley. Soccer can help get me in and I haven't decided if I really want to play in college yet."

Out of the mouth of babes. Mei considered sports, either track or soccer, as the means and a prestigious university as the end. Her priorities were sound and the pressure to perform was forever gone. She's an excellent student, always has been, and has the extracurricular credentials to excel at a top university. What she didn't realize is that sports is an unnecessary means to a very real end that will most likely be secured instead by a solid transcript, prestigious legal internships and an exemplary record of volunteering. It didn't matter what or how she played or who she played with or for. It mattered only that she played and that she was happy.

"The Plan 2.0" was set. Mei would return to practicing with her private trainer, Kodjo Gnaticko, shake off the rust and hopefully regain her previous dominating form. She would again play for Wootton and would consider club soccer. The latter wasn't a top priority and we both adamantly opposed playing for an authoritarian, but her former reputation and the Coyotes' past successes still resonated with coaches and she was immediately offered spots on four respectable teams: two ECNL, one EDP and one Girls Academy. Other coaches had invited her to practices and we had all summer to prepare for her senior year and, as part of "The Plan 2.0," ID camps across the country.

Kodjo's sessions were electrifying. Mei was running, dribbling and shooting on clouds, clouds filled with her perspiration and Maryland's humidity. The harder he worked her, the better she performed. She had grown 6 inches and gained 20 pounds since last working with Kodjo but was considerably more powerful and agile. She also had far more endurance than his other athletes and was compared to some of the college players who had worked with him over the summer. She laughed

200

and giggled again and was having the time of her life. Kodjo pushed his trainees physically but never yelled. Never. His critiques were sincere and accurate and we trusted him and his opinion completely, whether critical or complimentary.

Anticipation blossomed with the approach of Mei's first ID camp at the storied University of North Carolina. In addition to practices with Kodjo, she was running with her best friend and two-time Maryland state mile champion and playing or practicing soccer every day, scrimmaging with boys or playing 1-v-1 with other Division I college players. For the first time in over a year, she felt fast and strong and unbeatable.

ACT II. ACTION, COMPLICATIONS AND DILEMMA

We arrived at the Bill Koman Practice Complex at the University of North Carolina about an hour early. This particular camp, the College Bound Player's Academy or "CBPA," is the program's best summer camp. Coach Dorrance only holds a single ID camp every year and many of the attendees are invited and have already participated in the CBPA. It attracts talent from across the country as well as international players from several countries.

The first night consisted of mostly drills and ended with 3-v-3 scrimmages. Drills progressed in difficulty with coaches and North Carolina players watching, taking notes and talking between sessions, all to identify campers worthy of Dorrance's attention. Two teams of three played while two other teams waited along the back lines, spread out behind the goals. At the coach's discretion, one team would rush off the field while another ran on, keeping the ball and game continually moving. Mei and Katy, a tall and imposing Canadian youth national player, were on the same team and were dominating play with speed and power, respectively. The group's coach sent for Dorrance, who joined the onlooking crowd of parents cheering for what I considered the best and most aggressively physical high school soccer I've ever seen.

One of the two indelible plays from the camp happened that scrimmage. Mei's team had just sprinted onto the field and she immediately tackled and stole the ball, crossing it to her teammate on the far sideline. Katy moved up to the mid-field and Mei filled in behind as the ball was passed back to her. She then dribbled around a defender and passed the ball to Katy, who without hesitation lobbed it to the temporarily empty corner on the far side of the field. Mei raced passed the others, hurdled over an attempted slide tackle and in one motion landed and centered the ball to a crossing teammate for a dramatic tap-in. Parents from both teams screamed and applauded, the girls high-fived each other and all the watching coaches, including Dorrance, smiled and nodded with pleasure.

Mei walked on the clouds that night. She barely ate dinner and couldn't stop jabbering about the girls, coaches and scrimmage, about her confidence, her new Canadian friend and their dynamic duet. She was awestruck by Dorrance, that he singled out her group and she was giddy with excitement. I learned that the girls watched him like the politburo, monitoring his every move at the camp. "The Plan 2.0" was so far a smashing success!

The following day started with 1-v-1 drills. Mei's new group consisted of 16 hand-picked campers including Katy and most from her first day's group. A cone was placed in the middle of a circle and a ball atop the cone. Two campers entered the circle, an attacker with a ball and a defender protecting the cone. At the blow of a whistle, the attacker would attempt to dribble past the defender and to knock the ball off the cone with a shot. If a player missed, the roles reversed and a ball was quickly passed to the new attacker. Play then resumed until a winner was proclaimed.

This was Mei's jam. The Coyotes ran 1-v-1 drills almost every practice and Mei had worked with Kodjo to perfect moves and tight dribbling techniques. She loved 1-v-1 drills and regularly beat boys from elite club teams and even girls on Division I college teams. She was also dominating her group, undefeated during the practice period and in the competition, until the quarterfinal where a stalemate was decided by rock-paper-scissors. Competitions were limited to one minute and despite beating her opponent several times on the ball, she missed shooting at the cone.

The afternoon session was devoted entirely to 5-v-5 scrimmages. Mei's group was divided into two eight-person teams in a round-robin camp-wide competition. I arrived at the field late, coincidentally sitting down next to a parent of an opposing player. The mother surmised that Mei and Katy played on the same club team and was dumbfounded in learning that they had just met. Other parents chimed in, noticing the girls' symmetry of play, communication and advanced ball skills. I was both proud and humbled by the entire experience. Mei had busted her ass, risked years of hard work in two different sports and wasted a year and a half laboring in a sport she hated, but was now commanding attention in one of the most competitive high school soccer camps in the country, where that afternoon she was again undefeated. Yup, very proud indeed.

After a much-needed shower, nap and refueling of carbohydrates and electrolytes, we returned that evening for the 11-v-11 competitions. The camp was unusually crowded with parents and families lining the field. I dropped Mei off, parked in a distant lot and hiked back to the field only to discover that two teams, including Mei's, were taken indoors to play uninterrupted for Dorrance and the assistant coaches.

The Koman indoor facility is a modern athletic practice hub for all turf sports teams. It was funded in part through a generous $15,000,000 gift from Jim Koman, son of Bill Koman who played linebacker for the Tar Heels in the 1950s and later for three professional NFL teams. The facility was built primarily with football in mind, but not exclusively. The domed rectangular warehouse-like building has both natural and artificial lighting, climate control, a 120-yard turf field, football goalposts and a very noticeable 20-foot-tall cinderblock wall built specifically to Coach Dorrance's specifications for "living on the wall." Opposite the cinderblock wall are nine large retractable doors/walls, each separated by columns, that open like garage doors, expanding the playing surface to an outdoor turf field over twice the size. It's also physically connected to the most beautiful and best soccer-dedicated collegiate stadium in the country, Dorrance Field. To a female adolescent Division I soccer hopeful, it's the soccer Taj Mahal adorned in Carolina blue.

The girls were both excited and confused when directed to the facility. Some complained that coaches wouldn't see them play until others noticed Dorrance's absence from the practice fields. This fueled more speculation and anticipation. They talked quietly at first, following the crowd down the stairs and around a couple corners murmuring along the way. Mei couldn't remember who was leading or even how they found the building, only that everyone went silent when the door opened and they saw Dorrance standing along the sidelines.

The scrimmage had already started by the time I arrived. Mei was playing right wing in a 4-3-3 formation, Katy as right middle-back and field general, directing play and leading most builds from the back line. Mei was in a track meet, sprinting up and down the sideline chasing long passes and attacking mid-fielders. She later told me that one of her team's defenders said to the group, "If you get the ball, send it to the corner. Mei will get it!"

At some point, the other team had moved forward, pressing the middle of our defense and taking a contested shot that shanked off a defender. Katy recovered the loose ball and passed it to the left back who launched it to Appalachia, possibly even Tennessee. I watched the ball sail as Mei streaked through my peripheral vision and into focus. She alone was tracking the ball, at least initially as nobody thought she had a realistic chance of reaching it. A sole defender was also watching the ball and due to what I assume was shared disbelief, started jogging before suddenly sprinting to what everyone in the building, Mei included, saw as an inevitable collision.

A charge is defined as a "physical challenge against an opponent, usually using the shoulder and upper arm (which is kept close to the body)" in the official soccer rule book, the *Laws of the Game* issued by the International Football Association Board. Charges aren't necessarily fouls unless intentionally committed in a manner considered "careless, reckless or using excessive force." Moreover, "reckless" is defined as a "disregard to the danger to, or consequences for, an opponent." What constitutes a foul is, therefore, up to subjective interpretation, much like the strike zone in baseball.

Mei had just reached the ball, clipping it with the outside of her right foot when she was hit. I watched from behind as she leaned into the impending impact moments before it happened. The defender fell and Mei was thrown into the air, hitting the turf hard, bouncing and rolling twice with her head striking the ground both times. She lay motionless as assistant coaches sprinted to her side. My first terrified thought was concussion. Others arrived by her side and she still hadn't moved. Was she conscious? Should I run out there? Should someone call 911? How serious is it? What the hell is going on?

I ran up the sideline to get a better view and was relieved to see movement. She was still lying on her side but was clasping her knee. After an eternity, she slowly rolled to her back and was helped to her feet before collapsing with her first step. The coaches again helped her up and this time she carefully and gingerly limped to the sideline refusing to be carried. The trainer had been called so she sat down on the turf as Dorrance approached. She had an awkward forced smile on her face and was downplaying the pain, I could tell, and although she never cried, I could see the anguish in her face as her last chance for stardom dangled from her sunken shoulders.

I don't remember much else from that evening. Visions from the scrimmage and the impact are still vivid, so are the feelings of helplessness and disbelief. I was thoroughly distraught and told myself to stay strong for her, to be positive and downplay the significance, to embrace an unknown that was as much hopeful as it was wretched. I couldn't let her see my despair for fear of her own.

The trainer provided reason for tempered enthusiasm. The knee was too sore for a comprehensive exam, but the preliminary assessment suggested the anterior cruciate ligament or "ACL" was intact. She was guarded in her assessment, however, and warned that well-developed hamstrings, the biceps femoris, semitendinosus and semimembranosus muscles on the back side of the upper leg can somewhat compensate for a torn ACL. She was nevertheless optimistic and asked that we return the following morning for a second evaluation. Her diagnosis didn't change, but Mei's mood did because Dorrance called my cell and invited us to lunch.

We met outside a brunch restaurant close to our hotel and the athletic complex. Dorrance is well recognized in the city, naturally, and was bristling with UNC branding so it wasn't a surprise to find him speaking with a local fan or to be recognized by the restaurant staff. I've lived and worked in communities with famous coaches, most notably Mike Leach,

Chapter 10

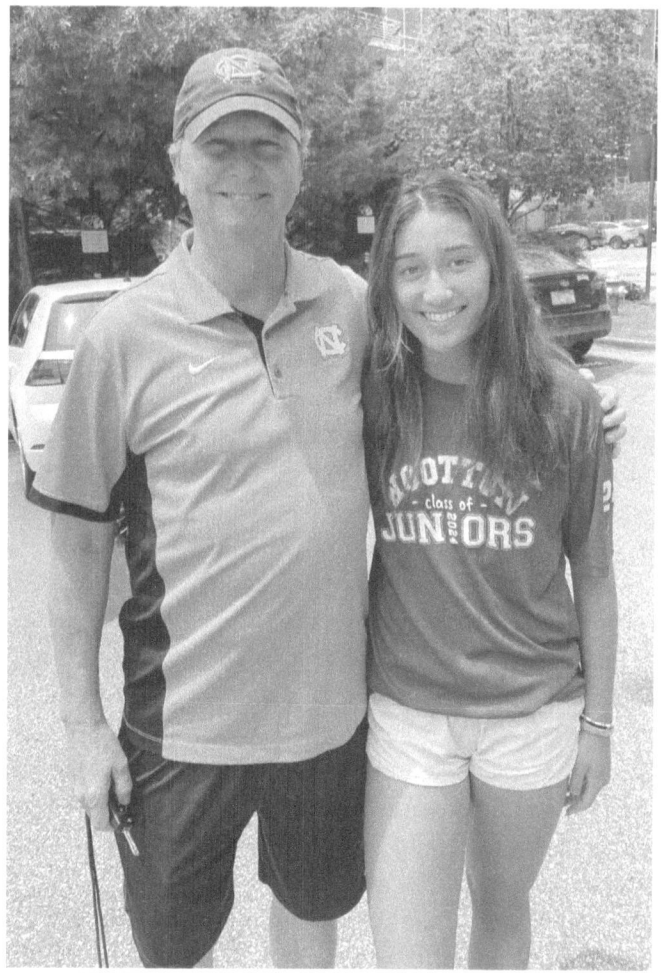

Coach Dorrance (left) with Meilani, July 20, 2023. Courtesy of the author.

the quirky, grandiose and larger-than-life football coach famous for the "Air Raid" offense, pirates and hilariously blunt interviews. Dorrance is the anti-Leach in many ways, highly affable and welcoming. He attracts attention yet never seems to crave it and, despite always having something to say, is incredibly attentive to others. In case you're wondering, no, I never attended UNC and until interviewing him, we had never spoken or even met. He's just very nice and highly personable. The kind of guy you want for a neighbor.

His staff and several players were also dining with us, but at a different table. Dorrance greeted them as we walked past and sat down immediately across from Mei. Aside from menu and other small talk, he spoke to her exclusively, asking questions about her playing and running experience, about training for both sports and past teams, about positions and positioning. He reviewed his coaching style and program and discussed specific players, name dropping several famous professionals whom he coached at UNC or on the USWNT. They discovered a mutual connection, the legendary Mia Hamm with 158 international goals, second only to Abby Wambach, and laughed over Mia's approach for marking players on set pieces: grabbing their shorts. He asked about her grades, about favorite books and classes, about a future major and about her inspirations and aspirations. He was recruiting her and she had no idea.

At the end of the meal, five or six coaches and players introduced themselves before leaving. She had met most of them during camp and some inquired how she was feeling and about the injury. They complimented her performance, noting her speed and competitiveness and, in an act of foreshadowing, offered to stay in touch. They were kind gestures, somewhat rehearsed, but sincere enough to mesmerize my awestruck daughter. In a kind, calm and confidently assuring voice, Dorrance then extended an offer to join the team.

Act III. Climax and Denouement

The long drive home was mostly upbeat. We share an affection for classic rock-n-roll and spent most of the drive singing songs by Creedence Clearwater Revival, the Kinks and Otis Redding when she wasn't sleeping. We were lucky to get an appointment with an orthopedist two days later who provided a similarly vague diagnosis and ordered an MRI. It was Friday and we had to wait until the following Wednesday before discussing the results. Everything had happened so quickly, the camp drills, competitions and scrimmages, the injury, the lunch and offer, the optimistic drive home and the orthopedist appointment filled with anxiety. Her emotions were riding a never-ending roller coaster and I could

Chapter 10

see the apprehension in her face when we turned on the computer and joined the telemedicine meeting. She desperately needed good news.

The doctor wasted no time. Mei tore her ACL. She also suffered a substantial contusion to the lateral condyle of her right femur and tears to the lateral meniscus and the posterior synovial membrane, resulting in a Baker or popliteal cyst behind the knee and synovial fluid leakage alongside the outer quadriceps muscle, the vastus lateralis. The meniscus could be easily repaired and the minor membrane tear would resolve with time, but surgery to repair the ACL and the following physical therapy would require 10 to 12 months for full recovery, assuming she exerted maximum effort.

It was over.

Years of hard work, of love and joy, of exultation and elation all vanished in an instant. The emotional roller coaster had come to an end, leaving Mei in an existential crisis. She would likely never play a college sport or leverage her talent in applications to Ivy League or other top-tier universities. All the hard work, the groggy early morning runs, the suffocating intervals on dark empty tracks, the pounding from defenders, the Kodjo sessions in blistering heat, the never-ending challenges from the bully coven, the obnoxious and callous parents, the frustrating, annoying and sometimes abusive coaches, the inspiring and devoted coaches, the never-ending ankle sprains, the cyclical sessions with physical therapists, the dozens of medals, ribbons, trophies and banners, the wins and goals were all for naught.

Or were they?

The news was indeed tragic, maybe not in the grand scheme of life but in the youthful eyes of an accomplished student athlete with a type-A personality and aspirations of grandeur, it was Sophoclean. Mei suddenly rose from the chair and walked out of the room. The orthopedist was still talking, unaware of gravity. Mei returned after a couple minutes with swollen eyes and flushed cheeks. She was fighting to maintain composure and clearly wanted no eye contact so I turned away, giving her the emotional space to absorb the orthopedist's a good-intentioned yet meaningless ramble.

PLOT TWISTS

A few days had passed before Mei would talk about it. She had always been an athlete, a hypercompetitive two-sport wonder who probably could have excelled at any number of sports, but now, in her mind, she was just a student. An excellent student, I assured her, and an athlete in repair, but an athlete nonetheless. It all fell on deaf ears. Nothing I nor the orthopedist said, no mention of studies or encouragement, could erase the truth. Her window of opportunity had closed. Fate apparently didn't want Mei competing in college, at least not via conventional or foreseen paths and as with Oedipus, her fate was revealed in stages: first in losing track to asthma and now soccer to injury. Her moment of realization was as precipitous as the impact itself, predictable in outcome only but not consequences. Mei alone would decide her fate, whether a tragic reversal of fortune and eureka moment of doom or an inspirational moment of salvation.

Adolescents infamously embrace the comfort and validation of hyperbole and Mei was wallowing in it. My normally gregarious daughter was uncharacteristically and understandably somber and although I trusted her resilience would eventually return, she had never faced anything definitive and I was genuinely worried. As with all adolescents, possibly with most girls, her self-esteem and identity were largely a product of her social perception. Her value as a person—in her mind but not in reality—was defined socially and she was avoiding the very people who could help her heal and deal. I felt she lacked perspective and eventually coerced her into a conversation.

I was blunt, purposefully composed and professional, recalling my days advising undergraduates struggling with courses and majors or graduate students failing their PhD qualifying exams. I reserved emotion only for reassurance and explained the realities of collegiate athletics, that only 2.4% of high school female athletes play Division I soccer and just 2.8% run track. The numbers are worse for boys with 1.3% and 1.9%, respectively, due to competition from other sports. I reassured her that she could still play soccer in college, although it would require a devotion I doubt she possessed. Our orthopedist was a skilled and highly recognized surgeon and Mei's drive is unquestionably strong so there was absolutely no doubt she'd approach her physical therapy with the

Chapter 10

intensity of a cage fighter, but she prioritized academics well over athletics and considered the alternative routes most traveled to Division I athletics, junior or community colleges antithetical to her academic goals. Far from arrogant, she understood her strengths and I applauded her pragmatism. I also provided some perspective using an unlikely source and a dear friend from the Coyotes.

Arya had followed Hyde to the Bethesda ECNL team and was a starting defensive back. The position fit her aggressive and irreverent personality better than forward and complemented her speed and competence on the ball. In fact, she was a standout at the position where she dominated forwards while playing for the dreaded Whitman high school team. As Coyotes, she and Mei were close and would hang out with a couple other non-blondes when the team would travel. Arya was a beast on the field and in the classroom and the two girls shared a common value of athletics and academics as well as a similar disdain for the bully coven. In fact, Arya was one of the girls who called Mei after the Nellie practice incident, saying, "Don't let those bitches get to you."

I had the utmost respect for Arya and her parents. The latter had survived previous relationships and had remarried to form a modern family with diverse racial, socioeconomic and cultural backgrounds similar to our own. The parents were both self-made people of influence, very successful in blue- and white-collar careers and had created what everyone perceived to be a happy and well-adjusted family, that is until Arya's older brother brutally murdered her father as she and her mother helplessly watched.

Details of the tragedy are irrelevant. It was horrendous, sudden and utterly unpredictable and its mentioning here serves a solitary purpose: to provide perspective. Mei's so-called tragedy paled in comparison. Arya lost a father. She lost a brother. She lost future memories and shared dreams and her life was irreparably assaulted. She was a victim not of fate but of a crime that robbed much more than a silly sport. Her challenges are easily more defeating and insurmountable than Mei's and they will be ever present, never forgotten and will haunt Arya and her mother in inconceivable ways that only survivors of such violence can appreciate.

This was Mei's reality check. We all need one, occasionally, and I'm no exception. In front of my keyboard sits a small cardboard box with a silver textured veneer that looks remarkably like the cross-section of a muscle, with an array of muscle fiber sizes as geometric shapes. Written on the lid is "When things get rough" next to a hand-drawn heart shape. Mei constructed it when she was 9 years old and filled it with a variety of affirmations, scraps of paper with an inspirational comment on one side—"I will always love you no matter what you do" or "If you do your best I will be proud of you no matter what"—and a congratulatory salutation on the other—"I'm so proud of you" or "I love you even more now." Yeah, it's a real tear jerker and it's my most prized possession.

CHAPTER 11

The ACL Problem

In the days following the news, I had repeated every affirmation in that box to Mei. She'd respond with, "You have to say that, you're my dad" or "I know" and return to her justifiably self-pitied state. Her reality check had its intended effect, however, and she gradually arose from the malaise and depression that often accompany injury. In fact, athletes frequently experience mood disturbance, self-esteem issues and even clinical depression with the more severe injuries. Such psychological changes are extremely well documented for neurological trauma victims but also for athletes who experience prolonged absence from play due to peripheral injuries that don't involve the head. Studies suggest that adolescent athletes are less likely to experience the psychological or mental health issues of their non-athletic peers, yet because they're adolescents, the risk for exacerbating these issues with injury is substantially greater than that of adult athletes. Simply put, injuries make the normally depressed teenager much more depressed.

Concussions have attracted substantial media attention over the last couple decades and for good reason. These injuries can have lasting and fatal consequences, although the frequency of concussions is relatively low when compared to limb injuries, especially in soccer. I'll also add that the vast majority of soccer concussions result from head-to-head and head-to-ground contact rather than from actually heading the ball. Notwithstanding, the relative risk for long-term absence due to a concussion is minimal compared to the much more common limb injuries and especially ACL tears. I don't mean to downplay the significance of a concussion or to suggest that it's somehow less concerning than limb injuries because it's not. However, I am suggesting that limb injuries and especially ACL tears have received insufficient attention over the years despite a mountain of evidence documenting the risks and long-term consequences they pose. In fact, ACL tears are among the most common debilitating injury for any sport and occur at a disturbingly high frequency in female soccer players of all ages.

The high frequency of ACL injuries was first noted in the early 1990s and by the decade's end, several review articles had been published in medical journals. Most if not all of these had noted a difference in the injury rates among men and women, a trend that has worsened over time. In fact, rates appear to have declined for men and boys, but have risen for women and girls, producing a three- to six-fold sex difference depending on the study. Women generally experience higher injury rates regardless of insult, but the ACL discrepancy is unprecedented.

Lower-limb injuries are the most common in soccer with ankle injuries leading the pack at approximately 1 for every 1,000 "exposure" hours of time practicing or competing. Knee, hamstring and hip injuries occur less frequently at rates of 0.6, 0.2 and 0.15 for every 1,000 hours. These approximations were calculated from several studies and reflect general averages rather than rates for any specific team, age group or geography, yet they're surprisingly consistent. The ACL injury rate is a subset of the general knee injury rate and is nearly identical to that of the hip. For an average elite club soccer team, an ECNL girls team for example, with a roster of 25 that practices three times a week for two hours over an eight-month period with at least one game or additional practice each week, the ACL injury rate would predict over three ACL tears for the team's typical four years of high school.

These sobering numbers are finally attracting media attention and are casually referred to as the "ACL problem." The 2023 Women's World Cup highlighted the problem due to the extraordinary number of the world's best players being sidelined by ACL tears, players that if assembled into a single team would be the hands-down favorite to win the tournament. Players like Christine Press and Catarina Macario from the USWNT, England's Beth Mead and Leah Williamson, France's Marie-Antoinette Katoto and Delphine Cascarino, the Netherlands' Vivianne Miedema, Canada's Janine Beckie, Sweden's Hanna Glas, Germany's Giulia Gwinn and Denmark's Nadia Narim. Add a goalie and the cup is all but guaranteed.

Media outlets are also speculating causes like gender disparities, resource allocation and quality, early specialization, basic biology and playing surfaces with the expected non-committal ambiguity of a politician. A few, like *Real Sports with Bryant Gumble*, have waded into the debate more bravely, suggesting that a familiar foe, artificial turf, might be to blame or is at least a significant contributing factor. I applaud the reporting and the willingness to investigate, but the conclusions are contradicted by overwhelming evidence rather than conjecture and anecdotes.

Epidemiologists at the University of Southern California's Keck School of Medicine analyzed over 1.5 million records from the NCAA Injury Surveillance System (ISS) database.[1] This included almost 31 million "athletic exposures" defined as "1 student-athlete participating in 1 NCAA-sanctioned practice or competition in which the athlete was exposed to the possibility of athletic injury." The sheer enormity of their dataset required them to calculate injury rates normalized to athletic exposures rather than exposure hours so it's difficult to make direct comparisons to other studies with much more limited datasets, but it really doesn't matter because the results were highly conclusive: grass, not turf, is more dangerous.

Across all NCAA divisions, the injury rates on turf and grass were nearly identical in match play but were almost nine times higher on grass during practice. Injury rates on grass were also higher during match play for Division II and III schools, but only when these data were analyzed independently. Data from women likely skewed the results as women were 11 times more likely to be injured on grass than turf whereas men were only 3 times more likely. The authors rightly concluded that soccer players of both sex experience a higher risk of an ACL injury when practicing on grass, although this risk does not transition to match play where contact injuries occur more frequently. In fact, most ACL injuries occurred during match play, suggesting that the more aggressive play compensates for any difference in playing surface.

Several questions remain unanswered. For example, how do multiple stratifying factors like previous injuries, type of turf, contact versus non-contact injuries, shoe type, playing conditions and athlete fatigue affect the results? Injury prevention programs have been demonstrated to reduce the number of ACL tears in soccer players by 22 to 40%, depending on the study. Exercise-based programs were the most effective and dropped injuries by 41 to 59% when both sexes were analyzed and by 45% for just women. It's doubtful, however, that including athletes who previously participated in such programs could have biased the results of the USC study because real-world rather than controlled studies indicate that prevention programs are rarely utilized and when they are employed, they only reduce injury rates by 13%. Thus, the presumption that playing on turf is more likely to result in an ACL tear is patently false. Coincidentally, a meta-analysis of prevention studies rated most of them as "low quality," although those that focused on lower-limb alignment were the most effective. This brings us to what I believe is the most compelling explanation for differences in ACL injury rates between the sexes: biology.

The knee joint aligns the upper leg bone or femur to the lower leg bone or tibia. The tibia is joined laterally to the fibula, and this three-bone complex is woven together primarily by five ligaments: medial and lateral collateral ligaments on the sides of the knee, the patellar ligament in front and the anterior and posterior cruciate ligaments in the middle. The ACL connects the front top of the tibia to the back of the femur whereas the posterior is oriented in the opposite direction, forming an "X."

Each ligament functions like a fairly taut spring, expanding slightly as the knee joint bends and rotates during movement. If the joint bends too far, the springs are similarly stretched too far and can snap or detach slightly from their insertion sites on the bone. ACL tears are usually stretches rather than complete tears, but the damaged ligament is incapable of recoiling and requires surgery to be repaired, usually with a small graft from the patellar ligament.

The ACL Problem

Proper alignment of the femur to tibia is defined by the Q-angle. If you remember your basic geometry, this is the angle formed by the leg and hypotenuse of a right triangle if its base ran parallel to the pelvis. To envision this, make an "L" with the thumb and forefinger on your left hand. Now place your hand over your right thigh with your finger pointing to your knee. The imaginary line connecting the tip of your finger to the end of your thumb forms the Q-angle. In men, this is normally about 12° with the leg extended whereas in women it's 50% larger at 18° and can sometimes be much larger. This is because the hip girdle widens when girls experience puberty, pushing the base of the triangle or tip of the thumb out.

A valgus alignment of the femur and tibia is often referred to as "knock-knee" and occurs more frequently in women than men due to the higher Q-angle. Men, by contrast, are more prone to having a varus or "bow-legged" alignment. Neither valgus nor varus alignments are normal, although the average woman's alignment is slightly valgus and this appears to heighten the risk for ACL injuries.

Hundreds of studies have documented sexual dimorphism in knee structure. These historically investigated gross anatomical differences in cadavers or in living subjects as they walked, hopped or jumped using rudimentary techniques like motion capture imaging. This is contrasted by the most modern kinematic studies using MRI to identify the exact ligament attachment sites and dynamic biplane radiography to image moving joints in real time. The latter uses X-rays to construct three-dimensional images with extreme resolutions, typically below a single millimeter and 1° of rotation, and can be used to quantify how each bone and ligament moves or transforms during exercise. The methodology is being used to evaluate the success of novel surgical procedures, to improve physical therapy and, in addition, to interrogate the ACL problem.

One particular study performed at the University of Pittsburgh's Freddie Fu Sports Medicine Center (reference shortly) and led by the center's founder himself, Dr. Freddie Fu, has confirmed what anatomists and exercise physiologists long suspected from less dynamic studies: the female knee is inherently prone to ACL injury under common athletic movements.[2]

Dr. Fu's study imaged the knees of collegiate athletes, all with typical knee structures for their sexes, while they performed a variety of dynamic exercises. Sprinting, for example, was studied because it's common to most sports and drop jumps because they're used to screen and assess ACL injury risk. Single-leg hops with a 180° rotation are commonly used to test knee rotational strength and stability and were, therefore, studied as a representative return-to-sport assessment.

Compared to men, women in the study were found to have a lower knee adduction angle especially when running, which is a scientific way of saying that they landed knock-kneed, and their tibia bones were placed more laterally (to the outside). This increased the relative ACL elongation or the degree of stretch compared to itself, although peak elongation was the same for both sexes. This disparity indicates that a woman's ACL is closer to taut with less slack by virtue of the femur and tibia alignment. Studies by other groups documented additional sexual dimorphisms in the actual structure of the ACL and, big surprise, it's larger in men and boys. Stated scientifically, the length, bundle size and cross-sectional area of an average man's ACL are all significantly greater than those of a comparably sized woman, either by height or weight. Moreover, ACL structures start to differentiate in boys and girls during early adolescence and in accordance with similar changes in muscle and bone mass.

The ACL problem in women's sports is biologically based. Yes, I'm a biologist, at least fundamentally, and yes, I understand and am more apt to accept biological and natural explanations over artificial or cultural, but not without evidence, and the anatomical and biomechanical evidence supporting a biological explanation are abundant and reproducible. By contrast, the several competing hypotheses that have recently materialized are at best mildly supported by correlations and at worst simple conjecture. Most have also been attributed to differences in gendered social influences and playing environments often without any supporting evidence whatsoever while others, like variation in menstrual cycles, patriarchal shoe designs and a shared poor work ethic among the fairer sex, are Hail Marry attempts at logic and borderline offensive.

The ACL Problem

The male ACL is thicker, longer and stronger. It's also more elastic while the male knee is structured in a way that places less strain on the ACL during exercise. The muscles that stabilize the knee, those that control the hips, knees and ankles are also larger and stronger in postpubertal boys and men. Ignoring all this in favor of unsubstantiated hypotheses further risks girls' and women's health as we become distracted to the most obvious solution: *creating* gendered playing environments.

Gender social influences in sports are indeed a causative factor in the ACL problem. I propose, however, that this isn't because girls are treated different from boys but because they're treated the same. Most sports were developed by and for men with rules that reflect gender bias. Some sports, for example, tennis and lacrosse, have revised rules for women, and although these alternatives may be based on a past misogynistic belief that women were incapable, playing three- instead of five-set matches in tennis and eliminating checking from lacrosse creates a less physically demanding and thus safer playing environment for women.

No, I'm not advocating three-set limits to tennis and I'd love to normalize all rules of sport, but only if it improves the safety *and* quality of play. Note the emphasis on "and." Wrapping our kids in bubble wrap would probably eliminate most injuries from most sports, but who'd want to watch a team of miniature Michelin men waddle around a soccer pitch to a 0–0 tie? Adding a three-point line, a rule against hand-checking and a restricted area or "no charge zone" has revolutionized basketball by moving the game to the perimeter and eliminating much of the ankle-spraining and ACL-tearing physicality of the game. Baseball similarly instituted rules to reduce collisions with the catcher, requiring runners to slide on close plays at the plate and preventing catchers from intentionally blocking it. It's high time that soccer did something similar.

Two proposed rule changes have the potential to revolutionize girls' and women's soccer in a way that mirrors basketball. They would significantly reduce but not eliminate the intensity of physical play and, as a result, injury rates across the board. Remember that the intended goal is to improve safety *and* quality of play and these changes would create a faster and more technical game built upon speed and finesse rather than brutality. After all, the Beautiful Game shouldn't resemble a roller derby.

Chapter 11

Rule Change #1: Adopting Temporary Dismissals
Temporary dismissals in soccer are analogous to ice hockey's penalty box or rugby's sin bin where offending players are removed from play and cannot be substituted until a defined period ends. Lacrosse, field hockey, water polo and some more obscure sports, even roller derby, have also adopted similar time-out periods with great success. In fact, the Football Association or England Football, soccer's governing body in England, introduced sin bins during the 2016/2017 season for most levels of youth soccer. Although the original intent was to curb dissent and regulate decorum, it has since been used across Europe and even in the United States to curb the more serious offenses that fall short of receiving a red card.

According to the Football Association's statistics, 72% of players, 77% of managers and coaches and 84% of referees voted to continue the pilot program and it was officially adopted in 2019. The initial program had an immediate effect, reducing the number of incidents by 38% and by inspiring teammates to police one another for obvious reasons: getting sin binned hurts the team. The Union of European Football Associations experimented extensively with sin bins for various yellow card offenses and reports similar changes to player attitudes and aggressive play, all of which has inspired IFAB to officially adopt temporary dismissal guidelines to the *Laws of the Game*. Unfortunately, guidelines aren't rules unless adopted by specific leagues, which is exactly what I advocate.

Everyone should admit that yellow cards are meaningless. I've seen youth players of all ages delight in receiving them and many referees are reluctant to use them precisely because the cards aren't respected. Applying temporary dismissals, however, for every yellow card would send a crystal-clear message to offenders and non-offenders alike: knock it off. It would halt the progressive escalation of aggression and fouls that commonly occur and often lead to violent collisions and injuries. The United States, unlike Europe, has been slow to adopt or even consider sin binning, yet I'm not alone in advocating it. Youth and college coaches alike have privately admitted to supporting sin bins largely because they believe it would prevent injuries, possibly their most significant concern. US Soccer uses IFAB rules and could presumably employ the tool immediately. They've even experimented with it in select tournaments, although for limited offenses—simulation (feigning/exaggerating fouls—aka flopping), deliberate delays, dissent and flagrant defensive tactics like pulling, holding or intentional handballs—but have expressed zero desire to adopt it nationwide at any level. The NCAA is worse and doesn't appear to have ever considered it.

Rule Change #2: Clearly Define Legal and Illegal Charges

Most injuries result from charges, and illegal charges are by definition ambiguously defined. Remember that a charge is officially defined as a "physical challenge against an opponent, usually using the shoulder and upper arm (which is kept close to the body)." It is defined as a foul if performed in a manner considered to be "careless, reckless or using excessive force," with reckless being defined as a "disregard to the danger to, or consequences for, an opponent," but what constitutes a "danger" or "excessive" and how is "disregard" to be interpreted? Are consequences demonstrated by outcomes alone? More simply put, does someone have to get injured before a foul is called, and if not, how in the world is a referee to predict consequences? Aside from employing actuaries as referees, it might be better to remove the ambiguity and clearly define what is and isn't allowed.

Defenders have a right to attack the ball but not an opposing player, and although playing the ball instead of the player can, under unique circumstances, still be considered "careless, reckless or using excessive force," eliminating intentional plays on the player would alleviate most high-velocity and high-impact collisions. A simple revision to the charging rule that specifically requires defenders to contact the ball before contacting an opposing player would remove much of the ambiguity and create a clearly defined criteria for distinguishing legal from illegal charges. The ambiguity of *playing* the ball would be replaced by first *contacting* the ball.

For example, legal charges could be defined as "a physical challenge against an opponent after first contacting the ball." Illegal charges, those not precluded by contacting the ball, would be immediately awarded a yellow card and temporary dismissal. A red card could also be given if the referee considered the offense a "serious foul," which is defined as "a tackle or challenge for the ball that endangers the safety of an opponent or uses excessive force or brutality." Such a change doesn't completely eliminate the ambiguity yet it clearly defines under what circumstances selective interpretation is employed: when contact isn't initiated with the ball and thus only when distinguishing yellow from red card fouls.

 I'd like to conclude by backtracking a bit and highlighting the absurdity of restricting these proposed rule changes to just the female game. The purpose of the changes isn't to create gendered playing environments per se but to reduce ACL and other injuries that result from overly aggressive play and high-impact collisions. Anyone familiar with both men's and women's soccer knows that the men's game is more technical and the women's more physical. It's counterintuitive but true. These changes, if judiciously implemented, could benefit everyone equally, and although they wouldn't affect non-contact ACL injury rates, 41% in male versus 53% in female high school athletes according to one recent study, they would seriously dent the primary cause of all low extremity injuries for both sexes: collisions.

Chapter 12

Postgame

The "IT," the cliché cited *ad nauseam* in every sports biography and even in chapter 2 of this very book, that special thing separating gifted athletes from other child athletes is no longer unknown and undefined. As with modern art, the amorphic nature of anything becomes more recognizable with familiarity. Pablo Picasso, Salvador Dali and especially Marcel Duchamp all embraced amorphic images in their work, yet the more we see and are moved by their work, the less foreign these objects appear. I am likewise and still starstruck by Meilani's IT, although IT no longer eludes me.

A personal favorite is Duchamp's *Nude Descending a Staircase*, an earth tone cubist painting of an anthropomorphic image gliding down stairs. The painting and Duchamp were heavily inspired by stop-motion photography and, as Duchamp described, "chronophotographs" of humans and animals in motion. The photographs and Duchamp's painting, one of a few that mimicked this technique, replicated dynamic motion with overlapping static images. With *Nude*, this was of a woman, although I challenge readers to decide for themselves whether the image appears more feminine or masculine. I used the image to introduce lectures on sexual ambiguities and for years my classes were always evenly split with some attributing circular hips to the feminine while others considered the rectangular chest masculine. Surprisingly few students

CHAPTER 12

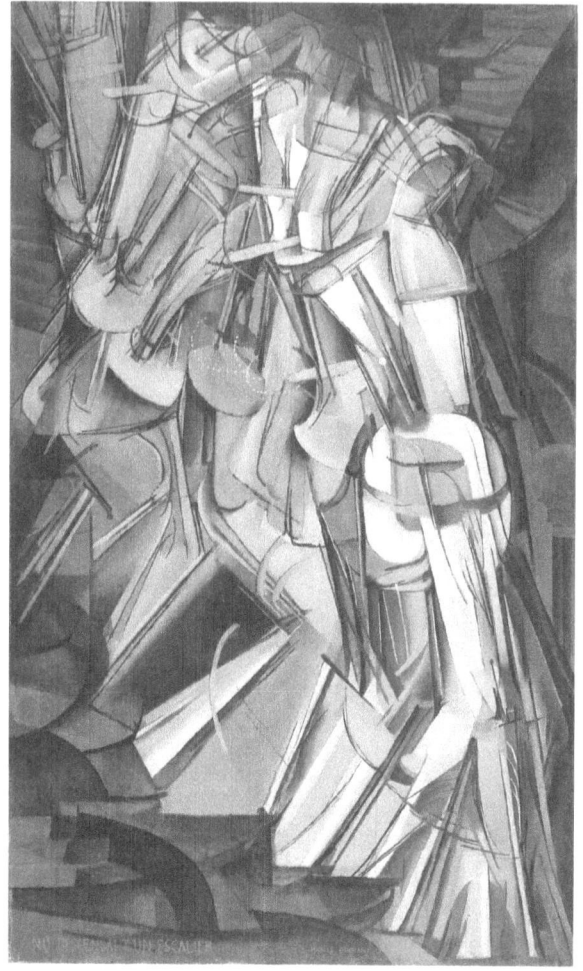

Nude Descending a Staircase, No. 2, Marcel Duchamp, 1912. Philadelphia Museum of Art, Philadelphia, Pennsylvania, USA.

immediately recognized the human form at first glance yet were unable to un-see it after hearing the painting's title.

There's nothing amorphic about Meilani's speed. She's fast and has outstanding endurance. She also commands a soccer ball better than most people can manipulate writing utensils or use cutlery and her reactions are just as innately reflexive. Her specific IT isn't athleticism, however, or any singular aspect of running or soccer nor the gestalt of many. What makes Meilani special in track and soccer or any sport she chooses to play, her IT, is a hyper-competitiveness.

She uses IT to beat my butt in Scrabble, to embarrass her brother in Ping-Pong, to frustrate my wife in arguments, to excel academically and, hopefully, to win at life. I don't know what role sports will play in her future or even if she'll continue to play in college, especially given the nature of her injury and its unfortunate timing, but I do know IT will help her to fully recover as IT has in the past. She may have had IT from the beginning, but sports, both individual and team, helped mold IT into more than just winning races and scoring goals, more than staying physically and mentally healthy, more than championing bullies, bad weather, abusive coaches and obnoxious parents and grandparents. IT milked the most of the positive experiences and found motivation and fortitude in the negative. IT ensured that all of these experiences were overwhelmingly enriching. Collectively, IT and sports have helped define who she is and who she will always be as a person, something I can't describe without getting emotional. I am so incredibly proud of her and who she has become and I will be forever grateful for the shared experiences we've had running and practicing together, however humiliating it was for me personally.

I started this book with a little self-reflection and admitted to living vicariously through my children's athletic accomplishments. If I'm being entirely honest, I'll further admit that my intrusions extend well beyond sports and that the emotional connection is rooted in not just a longing for innocence but in my own mortality. I don't want to control their lives or identity and I certainly don't want to interfere with their own experiences. I desire only to be a part of them, not all, but those consistent with forming a healthy parent/child relationship. It's a boundary I struggle to respect. Readers with older children are smiling and nodding right now and I'm sure some younger parents have the confidence to avoid such temptations, which the experienced among us would describe only as the hubris of ignorance.

So is living vicariously bad? Parents are by definition vicariously liable for their children, and although the degree of liability may wane as children transition into mature young adults, a child's accolades and condemnations largely result from what their parents do and don't do or, if you consider genetics, are or aren't. The problem is that the line separating responsibility from helicoptering is easily blurred as most involved parents soon realize. Those that don't could suffer the consequences of the many examples I describe and find themselves isolated along the sidelines, hated as the team's pariah or despised by their own children.

Experiencing joy vicariously through our children and their experiences is natural and good and altogether healthy. The temptation to control or get overinvolved is similarly natural, yet bad and altogether unhealthy. Balance and empathy are, therefore, key to parenting a child athlete. Every parent should be encouraged to get involved and to explore the limits of their involvement as long as boundaries and the children are respected. Parenting is not unlike coaching as both are, respectively, integral and important to the healthy mental and physical development of children. So cheer from the sidelines, embrace your new role as chauffeur, critique but don't criticize and if you have the time, knowledge and skill or the desire to acquire all three, coach. Just remember to do so for the children and not yourself.

MEILANI'S FINAL TAKE (17 YEARS OLD)

I was raised on sports, running in the cold and rain, forgoing parties and putting off homework for practice and studying late into the night after a workout. The drive to compete was always there even when it wasn't fun and when it hurt, was uncomfortable or embarrassing. I always assumed I would run or play soccer in college and it wasn't until I tore my ACL that my dream became just that, a dream. Soccer and track are much more than extracurricular activities, more than college application highlights and stocking stuffers. They define me, not completely, but they are ingrained in my personality, in my identity and who I am as a person. I am an athlete. I am also an intellectual and hope to someday become a lawyer or politician, yet the notion of moving forward in life without soccer or track, without competition and the extended team family, without such an integral part of who I am, was in the past unimaginable. Now, it's a little terrifying.

I was angry right after my surgery. I had overcome injuries and challenges in the past, yet this time there was a sense of permanence. How could I possibly play in college? I scooted downstairs on my butt and couldn't walk or sleep or even contemplate ever playing again at any level. Healing came slowly, recovery even slower and a hopeless feeling sunk to the bottom of my stomach. Family and friends offered encouragement, but their words were more irritating than inspiring, nothing more than painful reminders of my stolen dream. I didn't want to hear or talk about it, as if ignoring the problem made it disappear, and for the first time in my life, I felt defeated.

My parents worried. I'm sure they had never seen me in such despair, which is an unfamiliar emotion, but I admit to feeling lost. My dad pushed me to prioritize physical therapy. He told me that my physical health was more important than school, which led to arguments about skipping my assigned workouts at home. The important thing, the thing that I didn't immediately realize, is that he cared. He cared not about sports or grades but about me. He cared for my health and happiness and for my future. He cared so much that it felt wrong to not care myself. In an epiphany moment, I realized that physical therapy wasn't just preparing me for a future ID camp or a potential college tryout that, if I'm being perfectly honest, may never actually happen. It was preparing me for a future of early morning runs, of humiliating my brother in 1-on-1 or even teaching my future kids how to win a challenge. It was control and a return to a healthy body and a healthy mind.

I met him in a Starbucks after an early session with my therapist. We had been arguing about my commitment to therapy and I wasn't in the mood for a session that morning. He was still working on his laptop when I crutched over to his table and when he looked up, I leaned the crutches against a column and took a few unstable steps. It was my first time walking in several weeks. He smiled and tears welled in my eyes. We hugged, he cried, people stared and it was embarrassing. The few wobbly steps were a return not to but toward normality. They signified progress and justified the late-night stretching, squatting and lunging, the hours spinning on a stationary bike, the leg extensions and personalized therapy with Fumie, my miracle worker. Stairs were still difficult but not insurmountable and my knee was still swollen and scarred, but I could now imagine an end as well as a beginning. Quitting sports is not in my reality. I will always be running, always playing with a soccer ball and always passionate about play. It is, as my father says, my church.

Coach Dorrance's offer to play for the storied University of North Carolina women's soccer team was emotionally and spiritually gratifying. It validated years of hard work, sweat and lactic acid burning my legs and in a way is itself a minor dream fulfilled. It is also frustrating when I consider the "what ifs." I likely won't be playing in college or at any other highly competitive level ever again. This is my frustrating reality, but I'm fine with it. I'm fine because playing soccer and running track has given me so much more than the bragging rights of a college playing experience. I'm fine because they've taught me how to challenge myself, to push my body and my mind beyond what's remotely comfortable and to ignore that annoying inner voice constantly urging me to quit or take the shortcut. I'm fine because they've taught me how to lead, not through derision and denigration but through encouragement, support and persistence. I'm fine because they've taught me to respect myself, to earn and deserve respect from others and to never again tolerate abuse from authority.

Most of the abuses my friends and I experienced likely would have never happened if my teams, coaches and parents had adopted the Children's Bill of Rights in Sports. My coaches were too preoccupied with winning that they forwent any attention to individual player development beyond skills and strategy. I doubt they were aware of the bill, but if they were, they clearly ignored its focus on developing and mentoring players as people and not as objects. What's also clear is that strict adherence to the bill could only be achieved with a mechanism for anonymously reporting violations—laws are useless without police. There were so many times when I felt helpless and trapped. I was too scared to talk to my coaches, who were usually the problem, or to my parents, who could have made everything worse. Being weak or incapable was the worst of the Coyotes' sins so nobody publicly complained. A website, for example, for anonymous reporting or honest discussions of bullying and conflicts, with proper moderation by a parent or league representatives, would have made a world of difference. We were great, no doubt about it, but imagine how much better we could have been without the jealousy, fear and intimidation.

Changes to the game itself would also improve the playing experience, and although I would hate temporary dismissals, they'd actually improve the game, unlike yellow cards. I love the burning and proud feeling of getting a yellow card. It might sound bad, but it's a trophy. Coaches would proudly smirk, acknowledging their dirty teaching tactics, and my teammates' eyes became badges of honor to wear on my jersey. Yellow cards have no impact on the game other than telling me to hide my fouls better whereas temporary dismissals would immediately affect everyone and would, in my opinion, reinforce the technical skill of soccer rather than the violent and messy matches they've become.

Fouling is part of the game. Fouling secretly is also an artform and will never disappear from soccer even with temporary dismissals. Throwing elbows, pulling jerseys or shorts, clipping feet and, my personal favorite, digging sharpened fingernails into a particularly aggressive opponent's forearm are fundamental to winning challenges. Charges, on the other hand, can be physical assaults and evoke mixed emotions. The whole reason I likely won't be playing soccer in college is because of a violent and highly illegal charge, but I can't say I never did the same. If my coach told me to "get the ball," the integrity of my or my opponent's ACL never entered my mind. In fact, I missed most of my sophomore track season due to a bruised femur from an illegal charge that I initiated during a club soccer game. My father insists that this perfectly illustrates the need to better enforce charging fouls and I agree, but at the same time I fear the "babying down" of women's soccer.

A less physical game would clearly benefit speed and finesse players like myself, but would it change the game too much? How much is too much and at what cost? Women's sports are already portrayed as delicate substitutes to men's, which infuriates me. We are *not* less aggressive and I find it difficult to support anything, even a protective rule change, that could imply we can't handle the sport's physicality. Yes, I recognize the irony and my father equates this to the governance of clinical drug trials where oversight protects patients even from themselves, but I watched

Chapter 12

my brother play baseball and desperately wanted to play until I learned that girls played softball on a smaller field, with a larger and softer ball and underhand pitching. I then moved to Maryland, the nation's Mecca for lacrosse, and learned that girls' lacrosse is a no-contact sport unlike the gladiator-like boys' game. I understand the need for better regulation of charging fouls and I accept my own personal hypocrisy, but soccer cannot become the softball or lacrosse equivalents of the boys' game.

I'll conclude by addressing youth sports' peripheral participants, those with an inflated sense of importance—the parents and coaches—before offering some heartfelt advice to my peers. Parents, the game is for your kid and your kid only. Be there when they ask for help and be careful to critique but not criticize and always respect our boundaries because overstepping creates more issues. My dad always tried to help and I trust his intentions were honorable, but he sometimes confused critiques with criticisms and his opinions of coaches, even when spot-on and protective, were not always necessary. He generally let me figure things out for myself, but on occasion was a little too much, "overinvolved" maybe, and I lost my sense of independence.

There's a fine line between encouraging and forcing. I never wanted to quit soccer, but I knew several girls who did and who played feeling miserable. Parents have the unenviable job of determining whether kids want to quit because they don't enjoy the sport or whether something else like bullying or team dynamics is affecting them. They should encourage their kids to fight their own battles and push through the difficulties but also support what makes them happy and healthy, which can often lead to conflicting priorities. Yeah, I know it's hard, but isn't that parenting?

Coaches, the game is for your players and your players only. Your top priority should be to enforce love for the sport, not winning. Bad coaches chase athletes away, and rather than guiding and supporting their athletes, they seek to control them as if the kids were military automatons. Bad coaches have a self-serving focus on winning instead of creating winning players whereas good coaches embrace player development and understand that winning teams are composed of winning players and not a compilation of trophies. My next point should go without saying, but remember who you are. You, not a parent or league administrator, are the coach. You'll never please every parent, and pleasing some should never compromise the team or other players. Players and parents will come and go and to be honest, it's usually a relief when they leave. So let them go and remember: the game is for your players and your players only.

My final and most important message is to my fellow youth athlete. Playing a sport should not define who you are or what you're capable of becoming. Yes, it's part of you, a very important if not crucial, beloved and favorite part, but the complete you is and will become so much more! Do what you do because you enjoy it and play for yourself. Don't turn away from a challenge. Never give up. Be selfish, rude or nice, but play because you love the game, not for attention or even college scholarships. I know all too well the pain and depression from having my identity vaporized in a flash. I used to describe myself by track personal records, soccer goals scored or tournament victories, and it was unhealthy. Running and soccer will always be a part of my life and I especially crave them now that they're on hold. Temporarily losing sports forced me into self-reflection and I'm happy with who I am, with what sports has given me, which isn't wins or PRs. Sports isn't about winning but about learning to lose. It's about loving the game itself, about pushing your limits and thriving despite or even because of the pain. Sports isn't life, it's the inspiration to live.

Notes

Chapter 3: Body and Mind

1. Giulia S. Rossi and Patricia A. Wright, Does leaving water make fish smarter? Terrestrial exposure and exercise improve spatial learning in an amphibious fish, *Proceedings of the Royal Society, Biological Sciences* 288(1953):20210603, 2021.

2. Mohammad R. Islam et al., Exercise hormone irisin is a critical regulator of cognitive function, *Nature Metabolism* 3(8):1058–1070, 2021.

3. Joseph E. Donnelly et al., Physical activity, fitness, cognitive function, and academic achievement in children: A systematic review, *Medicine & Science in Sports & Exercise* 48(6):1197–1222, 2016.

4. UMass Memorial Health Center for Mindfulness, https://www.ummhealth.org/center-mindfulness.

Chapter 4: The Metamorphosis

1. Olivier Dupuy, Wafa Douzi, Dimitri Theurot, Laurent Bosquet, Benoit Dugué. An evidence-based approach for choosing post-exercise recovery techniques to reduce markers of muscle damage, soreness, fatigue, and inflammation: a systematic review with meta-analysis, *Frontiers in Physiology* 9:403, 2018.

2. Kim L. Bennell, K. L. Paterson, B. R. Metcalf, V. Duong, J. Eyles, J. Kasza, et al., Effect of intra-articular platelet-rich plasma vs placebo injection on pain and medial tibial cartilage volume in patients with knee osteoarthritis: The RESTORE randomized clinical trial, *JAMA* 326(20):2021–2030, 2021.

3. Liam D. A. Paget, G. Reurink, R. J. de Vos, A. Weir, M. H. Moen, S. M. A. Bierma-Zeinstra, et al., Effect of platelet-rich plasma injections vs placebo on ankle symptoms and function in patients with ankle osteoarthritis: A randomized clinical trial, *JAMA* 326(16):1595–1605, 2021.

4. Robert J. de Vos, A. Weir, H. T. van Schie, S. M. Bierma-Zeinstra, J. A. Verhaar, H. Weinans et al., Platelet-rich plasma injection for chronic Achilles tendinopathy: A randomized controlled trial, *JAMA* 303(2):144–149, 2010.

Chapter 5: Pink or Blue?

1. Jody L. Herman, Andrew R. Flores, and Kathryn K. O'Neill, How many adults and youth identify as transgender in the United States? The Williams Institute, UCLA, Los Angeles, 2022, https://williamsinstitute.law.ucla.edu/wp-content/uploads/Trans-Pop-Update-Jun-2022.pdf.

2. Paula Scanlan, Testimony before the House Judiciary Subcommittee on the Constitution and Limited Government, "The dangers and due process violations of 'gender-affirming care' for children," Independent Women's Forum, July 27, 2023, https://judiciary.house.gov/sites/evo-subsites/republicans-judiciary.house.gov/files/evo-media-document/scanlan-testimony.pdf; Forbes Breaking News, Former UPenn swimmer Paula Scanlan slams treatment for public opposition to swimming with Lia Thomas, YouTube, July 27, 2023, https://www.youtube.com/watch?v=6ltnVcb2zNM; Paula Scanlan, How the NCAA's transgender policies affect college sports, *The Penn Post*, April 9, 2024, https://thepennpost.com/2024/04/09/paula-scanlan-how-the-ncaas-transgender-policies-affect-college-sports/.

3. Helen Lewis, What the left refused to understand about women's sports: Female athletes said competing against trans women was an injustice, *The Athletic*, December 30, 2024.

4. NCAA, Participation policy for transgender student-athletes, https://www.ncaa.org/sports/2022/1/27/transgender-participation-policy.aspx.

CHAPTER 6: BOWLING BALLS, MEAT CLEAVERS AND CHAINSAWS

1. Aspen Institute, www.aspeninstitute.org.

2. Aspen Institute Project Play, Children's Bill of Rights in Sports, https://www.aspenprojectplay.org/childrens-rights-and-sports.

3. LiFE*sports*, https://lifesports.osu.edu.

4. Susan Crown Exchange, https://scefdn.org.

5. Anderson-Butcher, D. & Bates, S. (2022). National Coach Survey: Final Report. The Ohio State University LiFEsports Initiative, Columbus, OH. https://www.aspeninstitute.org/wp-content/uploads/2022/11/national-coach-survey-report-preliminary-analysis.pdf.

6. Diana Baumrind, Effects of authoritative parental control on child behavior, *Child Development* 37(4):887–907, 1966.

7. Diana Baumrind, Child care practices anteceding three patterns of preschool behavior, *Genetic Psychology Monographs* 75(1):43–88, 1967.

CHAPTER 7: TOTO, I'VE A FEELING WE'RE NOT IN IDAHO ANYMORE

1. Travis E. Dorsch and Jordan A. Blazo, Parenting Survey fall 2022, TeamSnap & Aspen Institute Project Play, 2022, https://www.aspeninstitute.org/wp-content/uploads/2023/02/TeamSnap-Project-Play-REPORT-v2.pdf.

CHAPTER 8: KILLING COYOTES

1. Molly Hensley-Clancy, FIFA invested in women and girls. Can it protect them? *The Washington Post*, July 27, 2023.

2. Meg Linehan, "This guy has a pattern": Amid institutional failure, former NWSL players accuse prominent coach of sexual coercion, *The Athletic*, September 30, 2021.

3. Sally Q. Yates. (2022) Report of the Independent Investigation to the U.S. Soccer Federation Concerning Allegations of Abusive Behavior and Sexual Misconduct in Women's Professional Soccer. King & Spalding, October 3. https://www.ussoccer.com/sally-q-yates-report-us-soccer.

4. Molly Hensley-Clancy, Where girls compete but men rule, *Washington Post*, November 18, 2022.

Chapter 9: Mount Rushmore

1. Amy He, Nicki Zink, and Ellyn Biggs, Fastest Growing Brands Report 2024, *Morning Consult*, December 2024.

2. Statista Research Department, Revenue of the WNBA 2022–2023, *Statista*, April 2024.

3. FIFA, Women's Football: Member Associations Survey Report 2023, https://digitalhub.fifa.com/m/28ed34bd888832a8/original/FIFA-Women-s-Football-MA-Survey-Report-2023.pdf.

Chapter 11: The ACL Problem

1. Mark Howard et al., Epidemiology of anterior cruciate ligament injury on natural grass versus artificial turf in soccer: 10-year data from the National Collegiate Athletic Association Injury Surveillance System, *Orthopaedic Journal of Sports Medicine* 8(7):2325967120934434, 2020.

2. Kyohei Nishida et al., Symmetry and sex differences in knee kinematics and ACL elongation in healthy collegiate athletes during high-impact activities revealed through dynamic biplane radiography, *Journal of Orthopaedic Research* 40:239–251, 2022.

Index

Note: Page references for figures are *italicized*.

abuse and bullying:
    girls' soccer and patriarchal culture, 142–44
    National Women's Soccer League investigation of, 141–43
    prevention of, 151–52.
    See also yates, sally
acne, 45–46, 68–70. *See also* isotretinoin
acupuncture, 61–63
Anterior cruciate ligament (ACL) injuries:
    knee joint alignments, 216–18
    rates of, 214–15
    rules to prevent, 220–22
    sexual dimorphism of, 214–15
Arlington Soccer Association, 126
Aspen Institute, 98, 99, 125, 126;
    National Survey of Children's Health, 85–86
    parenting survey, 128–30
    project Play, 99–100, 102, 104, 111. *See also* Childrens' Bill of Rights in Sports
Auriemma, Geno Coach, 158, 176–88;
    advice to players and parents, 180–81
    comparison to Coach Dorrance, 176–79, 185, 187
    concerns with youth basketball, 185–86
    evaluating talent, 180–81
    favored non-basketball credentials, 181–84
    name-image-likeness (nil), 176–79, 184, 187
    player biographies, 186–87
    recruiting for critical skills, 181
    scholarship criteria, 184–85
authoritarian coaching/parenting, 115–18, 143, 149, 175, 199
authoritative coaching/parenting, 5, 115–18, 175

Baumrind, Diana Dr.:
    parenting styles, 115
    parenting styles related to coaching, 116–18. *See also* authoritarian; authoritative; indulgent; neglectful

Childrens' Bill of Rights in Sports, 99–101, 152, 185, 226
chiropractic/chiropractors, 59–62
Colapinto, John:
    As Nature Made Him; The Boy who was Raised as a Girl by, 74–75

Dorrance, Anson Coach, 158–76, *206*;
    advice to players and parents, 175–76
    comparison to coach auriemma, 176–79, 185, 187
    concerns with youth soccer, 172–73
    evaluating talent, 161–67
    favored non-soccer credentials, 168–72
    player biographies, 173–74
    recruiting for critical skills, 167–68
    scholarship criteria, 171–72

Index

Elite Clubs National League (ECNL):
description and financials of, 126, 128–30
patriarchal culture of, 149–51

fibronectin-domain III containing 5 (FNDC5):
exercise and cognition, 25–28
neurodegenerative diseases, 28, 32–33. *See also* Irisin
Flanagan, Linda, 125–27

gender dysphoria, 73;
neural/brain development and, 76–77, 81
gender identity, 73–77;
brain structures, 76–77
natural basis of, 74–77
transgender athletes, 84–86
gender roles, 77
genotypic sex, 76, 80
classifying athletes by, 83, 85

Holy Trinity of coaching, 92, 93, 97, 99, 102–3;
coaching philosophies and, 106
scoring, 109–10
Hensley-Clancy, Molly, 130, 141, 149

indulgent coaching/parenting, 115–18, 167, 175
Irisin, 25–28
isotretinoin:
preventing side effects of, 68–70
trade names including Accutane ®, 68. *See also* acne

Kryptolebias marmoratus, mangrove killifish, 24–25

Linehan, Meg, 141, 151

Migeon, Claude, Dr., 81–82

nature *vs.* nurture, 78–79
neglectful coaching/parenting, 115–17
Nude Descending a Staircase by Marcel Duchamp, 221, *222*

Office of Alternative Medicine (OAM), 60–61

pain, 50–59;
active recovery, 55–57
compression garments, 55–56, 64, 66
cryotherapy, 55–57, 59, 69
DOMS, 53–58
massage and myofascial release, 55–58, 65
non-steroidal anti-inflammatory drugs (NSAIDS), 51–53, 55, 58
recommendations for management, 58–59
warm-up and cool-down routines, 54–55
physical activity and fitness:
benefiting cognition and learning, 24–25, 27–31
stress and anxiety, 33–37
mindfulness and mental training, 34–36
platelet-rich plasma (PRP) therapy:
treatment of tendinopathies, 50, 66–67. *See also* tendinopathies and shin splints
Puberty:
Athletic performance and, 83–84, 173, 215
body fat relationship, 46
bone mineralization, 47
boys *vs.* girls, 83–84
evolution of, 45–46
leptin, 47–48
transgender athletes and, 88–89

sexual development, 75–77, 80
sexual dimorphism in sports, 83–84

sexual orientation:
   animal studies, 75–77
   natural basis of, 73–75
Swyer syndrome, 81–82

tendinopathies and shin splints,
      62–67;
   recommendations to avoid, 64
   treatment approach, 65
   platelet-rich plasma (PRP) therapy,
      66–68
transgender athletes, 84–90

Yates, Sally, 141;
   U.S. Soccer Federation
      investigation, 141–43

www.ingramcontent.com/pod-product-compliance
Lightning Source LLC
LaVergne TN
LVHW090054080526
838200LV00082B/6